# CBS

## Quick Text Revision Series
## Important Text for Viva/MCQ's

# OTORHINOLARYNGOLOGY

**( For MBBS, BDS & Other Exams)**

**Second Edition**

# CBS

## Quick Text Revision Series
## Important Text for Viva/MCQ's

# OTORHINOLARYNGOLOGY

**( For MBBS, BDS & Other Exams)**

**Second Edition**


*Editor*

**Dr. M.S. Bhatia**
M.D., F.I.P., Dip. W.P.A., M.N.A.M.S.
Prof. & Head, Department of Psychiatry,
University College of Medical Sciences &
Guru Teg Bahadur Hospital,
Dilshad Garden, Delhi - 110 095 (India)

*Contributing Editor*

**Dr. (Mrs.) Nirmaljit Kaur** M.D.
Senior Specialist, Department of Microbiology,
Dr. R.M.L. Hospital,
New Delhi - 110 001 (India)


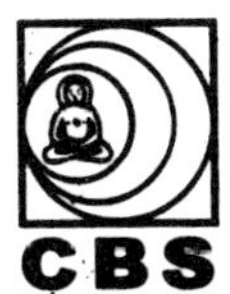



**CBS PUBLISHERS & DISTRIBUTORS PVT. LTD.**
New Delhi • Bangalore • Pune • Cochin • Chennai (India)

ISBN : 978-81-239-2195-2

First Edition : 2009
Second Edition : 2012



Published by Satish Kumar Jain and produced by V.K. Jain for
CBS Publishers & Distributors Pvt. Ltd.,
CBS Plaza, 4819/XI Prahlad Street, 24 Ansari Road, Daryaganj,
New Delhi - 110002, India. • Website: www.cbspd.com
e-mail: delhi@cbspd.com, cbspubs@airtelmail.in
Ph.: 23289259, 23266861, 23266867 • Fax: 011-23243014

*Branches:*

- ***Bengaluru:*** Seema House, 2975, 17th Cross, K.R. Road, Bansankari 2nd Stage, Bengaluru - 560070
  • Ph.: +91-80-26771678/79 • Fax: +91-80-26771680
  • E-mail: cbsbng@gmail.com, bangalore@cbspd.com
- ***Pune:*** Bhuruk Prestige, Sr. No. 52/12/2+1+3/2, Narhe, Haveli (Near Katraj-Dehu Road By-pass), Pune - 411051
  • Ph.: +91-20-64704058/59, 32342277 • E-mail: pune@cbspd.com
- ***Kochi:*** 36/14, Kalluvilakam, Lissie Hospital Road, Kochi - 682018, Kerala • Ph.: +91-484-4059061-65
  • Fax: +91-484-4059065 • E-mail: cochin@cbspd.com
- ***Chennai:*** 20, West Park Road, Shenoy Nagar, Chennai - 600030
  Ph.: +91-44-26260666, 26208620 • Fax: +91-44-42032115
  • E-mail: chennai@cbspd.com

*Printed at* :
J.S. Offset Printers, Delhi

*Dedicated to respected teachers*

*&*

*beloved students*

# PREFACE TO THE SECOND EDITION

Medical science is a rapidly advancing field. Its new allied branches are coming-up. In a competitive examination, more and more emphasis is being laid on these allied disciplines. But most of the standard textbooks of medicine have failed to devote adequate space to these new disciplines.

This New Quick Text Revision Series has been written with the aim to outline the major areas of various subjects.

Otorhinolaryngology includes Factual Data, Important Points for Viva/MCQ's, Anatomy of Ear, Commonest in Otorhinolaryngology, Physiology of Hearing, Disease of ear, Anatomy of Nose, Ear, Nose & Paranasal sinuses, Pharynx, Larynx, Oesophagus & Miscellaneous.

This book will also be useul for MBBS, BDS and other Entrance Examinations.

All suggestions for the modification of this book are welcome and will be duly acknowledged.

—Editors

# CONTENTS

# FACTUAL DATA ONE MUST KNOW

* In patients with hypercalcemia, approximately 80% of the patients have parathyroid adenomas, and 20% have diffuse hyperplasia. About 90% of the patients have **five** parathyroid glands, 5% of patients have **three,** and **3%** of patients have 1%.
* In **Presbyacusis** (seen in elderly over **60 years),** affects organ of corti, deafness is perceptive with increasing loss of tones above 1000 CPS.
* Juvenile Nasopharyngeal angiofibroma in commonest is **2-20 years** of age (mainly males).
* Head mirror is usually is forehead mirror **3.5 inches** in diameter, **0.75 inches** hole in centre and focal length of about **8-12 inches.**
* Malleus and Incus forms from **Ist arch** cartilage (Meckel's cartilage) and stapes from **2nd arch** cartilage (**Reichteric cartilage**) and otic capsule partly.
* **Mac Ewen's triangle** is landmark for mastoid antrum during mastoidectomy and antrum lies **15 mm** deep to surface.
* *Narrowest* part of facial canal is **4 mm** above stylomastoid foramen.
* Tuning fork have frequency of **256, 512, 1024** etc. and most useful is of **512 cps** (cycles per sec.)
* Middle ear structures have a resonant frequency of about **3000 Hz** the frequency around which human hearing is most acute.
* Curved tube of external ear is **2.5-3.0 cm** in length (outer 1/3 cartilaginous and inner 2/3 bony).
* Sphenoid sinuses are about **2 cm** in adults.
* Trachea extends from level of C6 to its bifurcation at T4. It is ***10-12 cm*** in length. It is flattened posteriorly. The upper ***6 rings*** are in neck and lower ***10-14 rings*** *are in thorax.*

* **20%** of mastoid bone is pneumatised.
* **128 double vibrations per second** tuning fork is not ideal testing of hearing.
* If a foreign body enters the bronchial tree, the right bronchi are more usually involved as it makes an angle with the vertical of about **25°.**
* With a bilateral meatal atresia normally accepted age for surgery is between **18 months to 2 years.**
* Time taken for complete recovery of nerve grafting may be from **18 months to 2 years** (1.5-2 year).
* Tympanic acitivity is like a biconcave disc, with height **15 mm**, A.P. length **13 mm**, transverse **6 mm** across upper part, **4 mm** across its lower part and **2 mm** across its centre.
* Eustachian tube is **3.75 cm** long in adults.
* Olfactory cells's central axons form about **20** olfactory nerves.
* Mitral and tuffed cells of olfactory bulb from **2nd** order neuron.
* In quiet respiration only **5 to 10%** of inspired air reaches the olfactory cleft while during sniffing upto **25%** reaches the olfactory bulb.
* During inspiration the negative pressure in the nasal cavity varies from **6 to 200 mm** of $H_2O$ in maximal inspiratory effort.
* Nasal cilia have an effective stroke and a recovery stroke and beat about **10 to 15 times per second.**
* Complete mucus-sheet of nose (mucosa) in cleared into the pharynx about **2 to 3 times** per hour.
* The temperature of the inspired air is man to **37°C** by the effective vessels radiating mechanism.
* Anatomic lack of access to the receptor cells of the **1st cranial** nerve is the most common cause of olfactory dysfunction (hyposmia or anosmia).
* The tonsils should be removed **6 to 8 weeks** following an attack of Quinsy (Peritonsillar abscess).

* The natural resonance of the external auditory canal (EAC) is ***3000 Hz.***

  The natural resonance of the middle ear ***800 Hz.***

  The natural resonance of the tympanic membrane (TM) is between ***800 and 1600 Hz.***

* The phase difference between the OW and RW is approximately **4dB.**

* Reflex decay is done at **500 Hz.** 10 dB above threshold, for 10 seconds. Abnormal decay is decay to less than 50% of the original amplitude in 10 seconds. That finding is indicative of probable nerve VIII or low brainstem lesion.

* Factors that can affect the **acoustic reflex** are :

  a. Conductive losses of **40 dB** for the reflex eliciting tone or as little as 10 dB for the probe ear.

  b. Cochlear hearing losses is greater than **70 dB.**

  c. VIII nerve lesions.

  d. Multiple stem lesions.

* Some basic rules of masking are :

  a. Masking is always presented by air conduction whether the testing is air conduction or bone conduction.

  b. Air conduction signals crossover at **50 dB.**

  c. Bone conduction signals crossover at **0 dB.**

  d. Crossover occurs to the bone conduction threshold, i.e., the cochlea (of the opposite ear).

  e. The purpose of masking is to eliminate the nontest ear from participating in the test. Masking should be done when :

     1. Testing air conduction whenever there is a difference between the level of the signal and the bone conduction of the nontest ear exceeding **50 dB.**

     2. Testing bone conduction anytime the unmasked audiogram shows an airborne gap.

  f. Bilateral **50 dB** air-borne gaps create some masking dilemma that requires special audiometric techniques.

* An air-borne gap of more than **50 dB** suggests discontinuity of ossicular chain.
* Even with otosclerotic lesions obliterating the oval window, it is unusual to find air-borne gaps of more than **50 dB.**
* The region of cochlea closest to the middle ear (promontary) is stimulated by sound in the **3000 to 50000 cycles per second** frequency range.
* Damage to the ossicular chain with an eardrum perforation usually causes a hearing loss of **30 to 50 dB.**
* Discontinuity of the hearing chain behind an intact tympanic membrane usually causes a conductive hearing loss of **55 to 65 dB.**
* In a acoustic neuroma diagnosis, a conduction delay of more than **4.6 msec** between waves I and V or 2.6 between I and III is significant.
* Although less specific **gallium 67** scanning is more helpful in following the progression of malignant otitis externa than is **technetium 99.**
* Approximately 50% of patients have a residual effusion **2 weeks after** the onset and treatment of acute otitis media.
* The true cord is **1.7 mm** thick. The most important laryngeal muscle for respiration and protection of airway is the posterior cricoarytenoid muscle, the only laryngeal muscle that abducts the vocal cords.
* In a newborn child, a subglottic lumen of less than **4 mm** is considered stenotic. A **5 mm** lumen is borderlined normal, and **6 mm** lumen is normal.
* A suprahyoid release during a tracheal resection allows approximately **5 cm** of mobilization.
* In patients with a chyle fistula, pressure should be applied unless the amount of leakage is more than **150 cc/day.** Open exploration with drainage and ligation of the thoracic duct is necessary for drainage in excess of 150 cc/day. A medium chain triglyceride is recommended for alimentation.
* The head and neck constitutes **9%** of total body surface area; the head is **7%** and the neck is **2%.**

* Thyroid cartilage begins to ossify at **25 years** and cricoid cartilage begins to ossify at **30 years** and both becomes bone by **65 years** of age.
* At the age of **6 yrs,** the larynx is opposite to C6 position.
* Radiotherapy is the treatment of choice for posterior **1/3rd** of Ca tongue.
* Development of human ear starts from **3rd week** of intrauterine life (IUL).
* The ratio of effective surface area of the pars tensa to the stapes foot plate is **14 : 1.**
* **Rinne's test** would be negative, if conductive hearing loss is > **15 to 20 dB.**
* **Weber's test** can be heard in affected ear where hearing loss is **only 5 dB.**
* A person with normal hearing should be able to hear 100% of words at about **5.5 meters**.
* Brainstem electrical response test becomes unreliable where the hearing loss is > **70 dB.**
* Electrocochleography and Brain stem electrical response tests are accurate to within **5 to 10 dB** of psychoacoustic threshold.
* Secretory otitis media (SOM) consists of conductive deafness of **30 to 40 dB** while CSOM deafness is **40 dB.**
* The process of pneumatization of the mastoid process begins few weeks prior to birth and completes at the end of **2nd year** of life.
* The corrective operation for pinnaplasty may be done from the age of **6 onwards**.
* The normally accepted age for bilateral meatal atresia surgery is between **18 months to 2 yrs.**
* Narrowest part of the facial canal is **4 mm** above the stylomastoid foramen. So, Bell's palsy starts at this area due to oedema of the facial canal, that presses the Facial nerve.
* Normal range for whispered voice is upto **12 ft** and conversation voice upto **20 to 40 ft.** in quiet surrounding.

* Thus, overall potential difference between Scala media and interior of hair cells is **160 mV.**
* Horizontal semicircular canal is in vertical plane when one is lying with a head-up tilt of **30°.**
* Cricoid cartilage ossifies at **30 years** of age.
* At the age of **6 years,** larynx is opposite C5 position.
* Olfactory cell's central axons form about **20 olfactory** nerves.
* Thyroid and cricoid cartilages become bone at **65 years** of age.
* Complete mucus sheet of nose is cleared into pharynx about **2-3 times** per hour.
* Capacity of frontal sinus is **7 ml**.
* 1 phon is the intensity level in decibels of **1000 Hz tone.**
* 1 sone corresponds to a loudness level of **40 phons**.
* Outer hair cells (UHCS) in inner ear are **about 20000.**
* Inside a hair cell is -150, -70 MV as compared to endolymph and perilymph respectively.
* 1 bel represents a **10 fold** change in sound energy.
* In benign nystagmus, there is a latent period of about **5s.**
* In inner ear, inner hair cells are in one row of about **3500** in number.
* Petrositis may follow a cortical mastoidectomy for mastoditis, usually **14-21 days later.**
* Three membranous semicircular canals communicate with utricle by **5 openings.**
* Retropharyngeal narrowing is **less than 3 mm** in older children.
* Prominent pyramidal lobe of thyroid is seen in **10%.**
* In xeroradiography, psammoma bodies in thyroid neoplasm is seen in **95%.**
* Development of ear starts from ***3rd week*** of intrauterine life.
* Adult average length of external acoustic meatus is ***24 mm.***
* External acoustic meatus outer 1/3rd cartilaginous portion is ***8 mm*** long and inner 2/3rd bony portion is ***16 mm long.***
* Adult average length of Eustachian tube is ***36 mm.***

* Eustachian tube outer 1/3 rd bony portion is ***12 mm*** long and inner 2/3rd cartilaginous portion is ***24 mm long.***
* Normal speech range is ***500 to 2000 Hz.***
* Hearing discomfort occurs at ***90 to 105 decibles*** (dB).
* Conversational or ordinary speaking voice which a normal ear should hear at **30 feet.**
* A normal conversation is heard over the spectrum of **500, 2000, 4000 cycles/second** (audiometry).
* The ratio of effective surface area of the pars tensa to the stapes footplate is **14 :1.**
* Eustachian tube obstruction may impair hearing (deafness exceeding **30-40** (db).
* CT scan combined with air-metogram can detect & outline cerebellopontine angle tumours **<1.5 cm** in diameter.
* Rinne's test will be -ve, if conductive hearing loss is **> 15-20 dB.**
* Weber's test can be heard in affected **ear** where hearing loss is only **5 dB.**
* A person with normal hearing should be able to hear 100% of words at about **5.5 metres.**
* A normal ear hears a whisper at **1.5 metres** (5 feet).
* Brainstem Electrical Responses test becomes unreliable where the hearing loss is **>70 dB.**
* Electrocochleography & Brainstem Electrical Responses tests are accurate to within **5-10 dB** of psychoacoustic threshold.
* Acoustic or stapedius reflex—excited by sound intensity of **90-105 dB.**
* When a sound of **70 dB** or more above threshold is presented to the ear—the stapedius muscle contracts.
* **4 months** old infant will only turn, however, to sounds made at 'ear level': he cannot locate sounds made above the head.
* In Rinne negative tuning-fork test, conductive hearing loss is **> 15-20 dB** (Rinne positive is normal).

* Secretory otitis media consist conductive deafness of **30-40 dB.** (CSOM deafness is **40 dB).**
* The most useful tuning-form for testing in early cases of conduction deafness is **256 Hz.**
* The most useful tuning-fork in estimating the amount of cochlear function is **1024 Hz.**
* Auricle is developed from **6 tubercles.**
* The process of pneumatization (air cell formation) of the mastoid process begins **few weeks** prior to birth & completes at the **end of second year of life.**
* Endolymph potassium is 150 mEq/1 & sodium is 1.5 mEq/l.
* Perilymph potassium is 6 mEq/l & sodium is 150 mEq/l.
* The corrective operation of pinnaplasty may be performed from the age of **6 onwards.**
* The normally accepted age for bilateral meatal atresia surgery is between **18 months to 2 years.**
* Normal saline at **38° (100°F)** is used as the irrigation solution for syringing.
* In diffuse otitis externa Merocel wick in the ear canal can be left in place for **2 or 3 days.**
* Regular attendance for local treatment lasting **3 or 4 weeks** is necessary for elimination of the otomycosis infection.
* Mumps cause sensorineural deafness on about **4th or 5th day** of the disease.
* In congenital syphilis the deafness is likely to commence in the **3rd, 4th or 5th decades,** where as in acquired disease the age of onset is always over **35 years** of age.
* If there is not recovery of sudden idiopathic deafness within **3 weeks,** it is unlikely to occur spontaneously.
* In hearing aids the range of amplification is usually from about **250 to 4000 Hz.**
* Significant hearing loss should ideally be diagnosed before the age of **1 year.**

* Adenoids may be associated with deafness.
* Acute tonsillitis may be associated with abdominal pain.
* Acute pharyngitis may accompany typhoid fever.
* Ulcerative gingivitis may be associated with malignancy of mouth and pharynx.
* Obstruction of the eustachian tube by an enlarged adenoid is a common cause of secretory otitis media (SOM).
* Male larynx increases in size at puberty.
* Cleft larynx is really a high TOF (Tracheo oesophageal fistula).
* The cricoid is the **only complete** ring in the whole respiratory tract.
* Laryngeal atresia is incompatible with life unless treatment is given at birth.
* In case of laryngeal obstruction, never give morphine.
* At birth the larynx is at the level of C2, 3, 4 position.
* Long standing oesophagitis may cause strictures.
* Commonest complications of oesophagoscopy is perforation of cricopharynx.
* Scleroderma of the oesophagus can cause difficulty in bolus transmission.
* Tracheostomy is done at the level of 3rd tracheal ring.
* Tonsils develop from 2nd pharyngeal pouch.
* Anterior 2/3rd of tongue is mobile while the posterior 1/3rd is fixed demarcation between the two is circumvallate papilla row in V-shaped manner.
* **Excessive salivation** is observed in :
  - — Peritonsillar abscess
  - — Malignancy
  - — Stomatitis.
* **Recognised causes of Macroglossia includes :**
  - — Haemangioma
  - — Lymphangioma.
  - — Myxoedema
  - — Acromegaly
  - — Pierre-Robin syndrome
  - — Tertiary syphilis
  - — Actinomycosis.

* Now-a-days, dissection method of tonsillectomy is the operation of choice.
* Following tonsillectomy operation reactionary haemorrhage occurs usually due to rise of blood pressure in the post-operative period.
* The disease causing **membranous lesions** in the pharynx includes :
  — Acute follicular tonsilitis.
  — Acute diptheric pharyngitis.
  — Vincent's angina.
  — Thrush (fungal infection).
  — Kissing disease/Glandular fever/Infectious mononucleosis.
  — Agranulocytic angina.
  — Acute streptococcal pharyngis
  — Keratosis pharyngitis.
* **Sleep-Apnea syndrome** is defined as 30 apneic episodes lasting 10 secs. or more in a 7 hrs. sleep. It is of 2 variety :
  a. Central sleep apnea (less common).
  b. Obstructive sleep apnea (most commonly seen).
* The anterior pillar of oropharynx consists of palatoglossus muscle.
* The posterior pillar consists of palatopharyngeus muscle.
* The normal vocal cord appear pearly white, owing to closely adherent epithelium + poor blood supply.
* **"Hot-potato" voice** is seen in pertonsillar abscess.
* Drugs causing **Parotid enlargement** includes :
  — Thiorueas : These stimulate flow and cause more viscous saliva.
  — Iodine.
  — Phenothiazines
* Tumours of the minor salivary glands are most likely to be malignant, with adenoid cystic carcinoma predominating.
* The AP soft tissue X-ray neck may show a narrowed subglottic airway (pencil sign) in laryngotracheobronchitis.
* In the adult unilateral vocal cord paralysis generally presents as horseness with a breathy character.

* Detection of radiolucent foreign bodies may be aided by inspiration expiration films that demonstrate air trapping distal to the obstructed segment.
* Foreign bodies in the oesophagus generally produce immediate symptoms of gagging and coughing.
* Haemangiomas the common on the face and neck, with most appearing at birth or by age 1.
* Severe gingivitis and stomatitis are frequent presenting symptoms of AIDS patients.
* Hairy leukòplakia occurring on the lateral border of the tongue is often an early finding in AIDS.
* When a sound of 70 dB or more above threshold is applied to ear the stapedius contracts.
* Rinne's tuning fork test is false negative in severe unilateral sensorineural deafness.
* Nystagmus provoked by the positional test is always an abnormal finding.
* The best and most formative method of inspection of ear is with an operating microscope.
* Tuning fork test provide a most reliable method of determining conductive or sensorineural type of deafness.
* **Weber's test** is important in false negative Rinne cases.
* If Rinne's test is negative in one ear and Weber's test is not lateralized to that ear it may indicate total deafness.
* Good hearing by bone conduction implies that cochlear and auditory nerve are functioning well.
* Brain stem electrical responses is now established as the **most reliable** audiological method of differentiating between cochlear and retrocochlear hearing losses.
* Autophony is due to eustachian tube blockage.
* Ear is fully developed at birth.
* Temporomandibular joint is a fairly common source of otalgia.

* The audiometric test which provides a quick objective measurement of the state of the middle ear is Acoustic impedence audiometry.
* The sense organ of hearing situated on the basilar membrane of the cochlea is organ of corti.
* That part of tympanic membrane bounded by the notch of Rivinus, deficient in fibrous tissue is known as **Shrapnell's membrane** (pars flaccida).
* **Weber's test** is very sensitive in conductive deafness.
* Disability of sensorineural deafness is more than that of conductive deafness.
* Normal saline at 38°C (100°F) is used in the irrigation solution for syringing.
* In diffuse otitis externa, **Merocel Wick** in the ear canal can be left in place for 2 or 3 days.
* **Blue drum** suggest cholesterol granuloma.
* Metabolic disease which may involve auricular cartilage is Gout.
* Keloids of the ear recur even after complete excision.
* Irritation of external auditory canal may induce cough.
* The ear lesion found in association with bronchiectasis and chronic sinusitis in young adults is keratosis obturans.
* Itching is prominent symptom in otomycosis.
* Circumscribed serous meningitis commonly occurs in the posterior cranial fossa.
* Hairline or bubbles visible through the T.M. is specifically diagnostic of acute non-suppurative otitis media.
* The characteristic feature of chronic salpingitis is retraction of the drumhead in whole or in part.
* A malignant polypus is often nodular, painful, friable and haemorrhagic.
* Cochlear lesions are far more likely to cause recruitment than are lesions of the acoustic nerve or central connections.
* Suppurative labyrinthitis cause severe vertigo.
* Audiogram and caloric test are normal in positional vertigo.

* A facial palsy complicating parotid tumour suggests malignancy.
* **Tumarkin** showed failure of middle ear cleft aeration due to eustachian tube dysfunctions.
* **Diamant** gave the theory of deficient pneumatisation of mastoid air cells due to congenital variation.
* Wittmaark established theory of deficient pneumatisation in mastoid air cells due to infantile otitis media.
* Clinically, **Mac Ewen's** triangle/Suprameatal triangle is palpated in the Cymba concha of the pinna.
* The **Place theory of Helmholtz** postulates that perception of pitch of sound depends upon the selective maximal vibratory action by a certain place along the basilar membrane.
* **Rutherford's telephone theory** considers that perilymph and basilar membrane are stimulated by every frequency of sound as in diaphragm of telephone. So, pitch perception is determined upon the number of times per second the fibres of auditory nerve discharge.
* The **Travelling wave theory of Bekesy** is the most accepted theory about hearing. According to this the points along the cochlea at which the travelling wave of sound reacts maximum vary with the frequency. The high tone is at basal coil and low tone at apical region.
* BERA (Brain stem Evoked Response Audiometry) is the most modern diagnostic test for acoustic neuroma.
* Surgical decompression of the VIIth CN (Facial nerve) is done when the ENG shows degeneration of 95% of nerve fibres.
* MRI is the **most important** imaging technique in recent times to diagnose the acoustic neuroma.
* **Evolved Response Audiometry** (ERA) is the **most recent** advancement in audiology which is more objective in diagnosis of cochlear and retro-cochlear lesions.
* Inadequate treatment in cases of ASOM often results in latent infection in the pneumatised **mastoid** or **"mastoid reservoir phenomenon"**. This is seen more often in penicillin resistant cases.

* **Tullio phenomenon** is the condition where a subject gets attacks of dizziness or vertigo by loud sounds. It can occur in patients of labyrinthine fistula.

* **Development of ear**

— Aurical—Develops from 6 tubercles (3 from 1st arch & 3 from 2nd arch) appear at about 4th week of IUL.

— **External auditory canal** : It has got two parts :

(i) Cartilaginous part—ectoderm of 1st visceral cleft.

(ii) Bony part — Os tympanum.

— **Tympanic membrane** : It has got 3 layer structure :

(i) Outer epithelial layer : ectodermal

(ii) Middle fibrous layer : mesodermal.

(iii) Inner mucosal layer : endodermal

— **Tympanic cavity and eustachian tube :**

— Endodermal develops from tubo tympanic recess.

— Ossicles : They are 3 in number :

(i) Malleus develops from mesoderm of 1st visceral arch or Meckel's cartilage.

(ii) Incus

(iii) Stapes It consists of following anatomical parts.

Head

Neck develops from mesoderm of 2nd visceral arch or Reichter's cartilage.

Crura.

Foot plate—develops from ottic capsule.

* Inner ear

Membranous labyrinth develops from ectoderm near hindbrain. Bony labyrinth develops from mesoderm around membranous labyrinth.

* The T.M. is almost horizonal in an infant but in an adult is placed obliquely in such a manner that its antero-inferior margin is in a deeper plane than its posterosuperior margin. It forms an angle of about **40° to 45°** with the anterior wall of external auditory canal.

* T.M. is divided into 2 parts :
  (i) Pars tensa—It has got all the 3 layers of T.M.
  (ii) Pars flaccida—It has also got 3 layers but middle layer is deficient.
* The T.M has 3 layers :
  Outer —epidermal layer.
  Middle — fibrous layer.
  Inner — mucosal layer.
* In infants, eustachian tube is more horizontal, wider and shorter, so infection reaches more easily to middle ear.
* 3 semicircular canals, horizontal, superior and posterior are set at right angles to one another.
* Sound travels at the rate of :
  **330 m/sec**— in air
  **1437 m/scc** — in water
* Sounds of increasing frequency have a shorter wave length. **256 Hz** means that tuning fork vibrates at **256 cycles/sec.**
* Threshold for normal hearing is 0dB. From a distance of 1 metre the sound intensity is :

| | | |
|---|---|---|
| Whisper | — | 30 dB |
| Normal talk | — | 40 dB |
| Shout | — | 90 dB |
| Discomfort | — | 120 dB |

* Hydraulic action : This action depends on the Areal ratio of the tympanic membrane and oval window. The ratio is about 14 : 1 (overall ratio is 1.3 x 14.1 = 18 :1)
  Resting potentials in cochlea

| | | |
|---|---|---|
| Scala Tympani | — | + 0mV |
| Scala Vestibuli | — | + 5 mV |
| Scala Media | — | + 80 mV |
| Hair Cells | — | -80 mV |

* The utricle maintains static equibrium and linear acceleration.

* The semicircular canals respond to angular acceleration.
* **Puretone audiometry** is basically a quantitative test and it tells us how much the deafness is present. It does not provide information regarding the nature of pathology and the site of the lesion.
* Grading of Audiograms.

| | | |
|---|---|---|
| Normal hearing level | — | 10 to 26 dB |
| Mild deafness | — | 27 to 40 dB |
| Moderate deafness | — | 41 to 55 dB |
| Moderate to severe deafness | — | 56 to 70 dB |
| Severe deafness | — | 71 to 90 dB |
| Profound deafness • | — | above 90 dB |

* The hearing level mentioned is the pure tone average of the hearing threshold level at 500, 1000, 2000 Hz only — since this is the frequency range of normal human speech.
* If the bone conduction level is normal (within say 15 dB to 20 dB H.L) but the air bone gap is 20 dB or more then the deafness is conductive in type.
* If the bone conduction level is more than 20 dB and if the air bone gap is 15 dB or lesser than the deafness is sensorineural in type.
* If the bone conduction level is worse (more) 20 dB and the air bone gap is 20 dB or more then the deafness is mixed in type.
* **Recruitment**

  — it is defined as a phenomenon observed in certain forms of deafness wherein the growth of loudness of sound of increasing intensity is greater than in normal ears.

  — It is suggestive of a cochlear (sensory) lesion.
* **Fowler's loudness Balance test.**

  — For demonstrating recruitment.

  Tone decay—to diagnose acoustic nerve deafness.

  Loudness discomfort level—nerve lesion patients may not experience any discomfort at any intensity.
* **Acoustic reflex decay or absence :** Suggests the presence of acoustic nerve lesion.

* **Electrocochleography :** Measures the electrical activity generated in cochlea in response to a click stimulus and useful in threshold estimation in children who cannot be tested by other means.
* **Brainstem electrical response** (non-invasive)-is the most reliable audiological method of differentiating between cochlear and retrocochlear hearing loss.

  Note : (i) It is unreliable if hearing loss > 70 dB.

  (ii) Normal pattern of waves maintained in cochlear deafness (Meniere's disease) and wave pattern altered in retrocochlear lesions (acoustic neuroma or cerebellopontine angle tumours).
* **Fitzerald-Hallpike test or Differentiate caloric test**
  - This test is conducted while patient lying on couch and head 30° above horizontal.
  - Irrigation of water with 7°C above and 7°C below body temperature — at 30°C and 44°C using a minimum of 250 ml each time (for about 40 seconds irrigated).
  - With nystagmus lasting for about 2 mts—fast component being towards the irrigated ear with the hot stimulus and in the opposite direction with cold.
  - Results or interpretation :
    a) Complete or incomplete canal paresis —lesion in peripheral vestibular apparatus.
    b) Directional preponderance of nystagmus— indicates dysfunction in vestibular potency.
  - Amplitude of the nystagmus reflexes the neural activity provoking it.
* **Electronystagmography (ENG) :**
  - ENG records eye movements and so nystagmus.
  - Nystagmus—saw tooth appearance.
  - Pendulum test—shows irregular tracing in cerebellar dysfunction.
  - Optokinetic nystagmus—asymmetry suggests central lesion.
  - Fistula test—detects circumscribed labyrinthitis.

— In typical fistula—shows nystagmus (diseased side) and slow movement (opposite side).

— Reversed fistula sign—slow component (diseased side). Labyrinthine fenestration procedure can produce a positive fistula test.

* Irrigation should be performed only when tympanic membrane is known to be intact. Following irrigation, the ear canal should be thoroughly dried (e.g. by instilling isopropyl alcohol or using a hair blow drier on pressure setting) to reduce the likehood of inducing external otitis.

* **Malignant otitis media** usually caused by pseudomonas, osteomyelitis begins in the floor of the ear canal and may extend into the middle fossa floor, the clivus and even the contralateral skull base.

* The patient with malignant otitis media usually presents with persistent foul smelling aural discharge, granulations in the ear canal, deep otalgia and progressive cranial nerve palsies involving nerve VI, VII, IX, X, XI or XII.

* Underwater diving represents even a greater barometric stress to the ear than flying.

* The **absolute contraindication** to diving is tympanic membrane perforation.

  **Note :** In newborn infants gram -ve enteric pathogens (E. coli etc) predominates.

* Bullae on tympanic membrane - Mycoplasma pneumoniae.

* Tympanocentesis is useful for :

  — otitis media in immunocompromised patients.

  — in neonates in whom gram-ve organisms are common.

  — in cases of persistent infection despite multiple courses of antibiotics.

* Myringotomy is reserved for patients with severe otalgia or when complications of otitis (e.g. mastoiditis, meningitis) have occurred.

* Common organisms causing CSOM include :
  — Pseudomonas aeruginosa.
  — Proteus species.
  — Staph. aureus.
  — Mixed anaerobic infections.
* The clinical hallmark of CSOM is purulent aural discharge.
* The definitive management of CSOM/COM is surgical in most cases.
* When mastoid air cells are involved by irreversible infection, they should be exenterated through mastoidectomy.
* If arises from haematogenous spread from ASOM, most commonly are H. inflenzae & S. pneumoniae.
* Some evidence suggests that this level of hearing loss may be stabilized by treatment with oral NaF (sodium fluoride) over prolonged period.

  Drugs should preferably be taken with meals to prevent gastric irritation.
* Haemorrhage behind an intact T.M. (haemotympanum) may follow blunt trauma or extreme barotrauma. Spontaneous resolution over several weeks in the usual course.
* Acute severe pain out or proportion to the physical findings may be due to herpes zoster oticus, especially when vesicles appear in the ear canal or concha.
* CSOM is usually not painful except during acute exacerbation.
* Persistent pain and discharge from the ear suggest osteomyelitis of the skull base or cancer.
* Repeated episodes of severe lancinating otalgia may occur in glossopharyngeal neuralgia. It responds well to microvascular decompression of the IX nerve.
* Infections and neoplasia that involve the orophaynx, hypopharynx and larynx frequently cause otalgia.
* Peristent tinnitus usually indicates the presence of sensory hearing loss.

* Intermittent periods of mild, high pitched tinnitus lasting for several minutes are common in normal hearing persons.
* To establish a definitive diagnosis of tinnitus a CT scan and vascular studies are often necessary.
* Thus vertigo is not just **"spinning"** but may present as a sense of tumbling, or falling forward or backward, or of the ground rolling beneath one's feet ("earthquake-like").
* The **Nylen-Barany manoeuvers** are intended to induce positioning nystagmus but are of limited use when the patient is able to visually fixate. This objection may be overcome either by placing + 2D lenses (Frensel glasses) over the eyes or by making observations in the dark by means of electronystagmographic recording.
* The **Fukuda test** in which the patient marches in place with eyes closed, is useful for detecting subtle defects. A positive response is observed when the patient rotates, usually toward the side cf the diseased labyrinth.
* Episodic vertigo resembling that of Meniere's syndrome but without accompanying auditory symptoms is known as recurrent vestibulopathy.
* One characteristic of neural hearing loss is deterioration of speech discrimination out of proportion to the decrease in pure tone thresholds. Another is auditory adaptation.
* Auditory evoked responses are useful in distinguishing cochlear from neural losses and may give insight into the site of lesion within the central pathways.
* Vertigo arising from central lesions tends to be more chronic and debilitating than that seen in labyrinthine disease.
* Most patient with multiple sclerosis suffer from episodic vertigo and chronic imbalance.
* **Goldenhar's syndrome**
  — Atretic external auditory canal, ossicles & anomalous (7th CN) facial nerve.
  — Congenital ocular dermoids.
  — Notching of upper eye lids.
  — Vertebral anomalies.

* **Wilder Vanck syndrome**
  - — Abducent (6th CN) Nerve palsy.
  - — Pre auricular sinuses and appendages.
  - — Fusion of cervical vertebrae.
  - — Perceptive deafness.
* **Crouzon's syndrome (Cranio-facial dysostosis)**
  - — Atretic external canal
  - — Fixed or deformed ossicles
  - — Normal facial nerve (7th CN).
  - — Exophthalmous.
  - — Divergent squint.
  - — Underdeveloped maxillae.
  - — Hypertelorism
  - — Parrot-beak nose
* **Dysplasia**

  a) **Scheibe dysplasia :**
  - — Sacculo-cochlear.
  - — Involves saccule and cochlea only.
  - — Bony and membranous labyrinth and utricle are normal.
  - — Stria vascularis is deformed
  - — Reissner's membrane is collapsed.
  - — Rudimentary organ of corti.
  - — Not associated with any other developmental anomaly.

  b) **Mondini-Alexander dysplasia :**
  - — Cochlea is reduced to 1.5 turns.
  - — Rudimentary organ of corti.
  - — Underdeveloped Vestibular structures.
  - — Diagnosed by Polytomography.

c) **Bing-Siebenmann dysplasia :**

— Bony labyrinth is fully developed.

— Membranous labyrinth is underdeveloped

— Often associated with Retinitis Pigmentosa.

d) **Michael dysplasia :**

— Total absence of both labyrinths are seen.

* Indications of **myringotomy** in acute otitis media (AOM)

— Not responding to treatment after 48 hrs.

— Patient is having agonising pain.

— Drum-red, bulged with a yellow area of impending perforation.

— Headache

— Vomiting

— Facial weakness

— Vertigo or giddiness

* **Indications of myringotomy** in secretory otitis media

— Eradication of septic focus.

— Steroids for 2 to 3 months be given.

— Antibiotic (not universally agreed).

— Patient develops sharp deterioration in hearing.

— Adhesion of the tympanic membrane with the middle ear mucosa for ossicles.

— Development of a silent perforation.

* **Function of Grommet :**

a) Aspiration and drainage of fluid

b) Provide aeration of the tympanic cavity.

* **Complications of Grommet insertion**

a) Tympanosclerosis

b) CSOM

c) Grommet pushed in middle ear cavity.

* **Characteristics of Adenoid facies**

a) Half open mouth
b) Expressionless face
c) Obliteration of nasolabial furrow
d) Pinched-up nose
e) Overcrowding of teeth
f) Protrusion of upper jaw
g) Recession of lower jaw
h) High arched palate.

* **Common microbes in ENT**

**a) Nose and Paranasal Sinuses**

— Streptococcus pneumoniae
— H. influenzae
— Gr. A. Streptococcus pyogenes
— Klebsiella
— Anaerobic streptococci.
— Staphylococcus aureus.

**b) External auditory canal**

— Pseudomonas aeruginosa.
— Staphylococcus aureus.
— Streptococcus pyogenes.
— Streptococcus pneumoniae
— H. influenzae (in children)

**c) Middle Ear**

— Streptococcus pneumoniae.
— H. influenzae
— Branhamella catarrhalis.
— Streptococcus pyogenes.
— Staph. aureus.
— Anaerobic streptococci.
— Bacteriodes.
— Gram negative bacilli.
— Mycobacterial tuberculosis.

**d) Throat**

— Gr. A Streptococcus pyogenes

— Corynebacterium diphtheriae

— Neisseria meningitidis/gonorrhoea.

— Vincent's disease

— Bordetella pertussis

— H. influenzae

* Indications of Laser therapy

1. Head and Neck :

— Warts, naevi, moles and tatoos.

2. Throat :

a) Pharynx :

— Lesions of buccal mucosa

e.g . Haemangioma

Lymphangioma

Hyperkeratotic lesions

Papilloma and Rhinosporidiosis.

— Tonsillectomy (both child and adult)

— Partial glossectomy

— Debulking of large tumour for paliation.

b) Larynx :

— Vocal nodules and polyps

— Hyperkeratotic lesions of vocal cords.

— Recurrent respiratory papilloma.

— Ca. in situ or T1 lesion of vocal cord.

— Verrucous Ca.

— Laryngeal web.

— Subglottic stenosis and haemangioma.

— Stripping of vocal cord.

— Biopsy

3. Nose :

— Rhinophyma
— Epistaxis.
— Inferior nasal turbinectomy
— Rhinosporidiosis
— Basal cell Ca. of skin
— Hereditary haemorrhagic telengiectasia.
— Choanal atresia
— Recurrent inverted papilloma.

4. Ear :

a. External ear :

— Lesions of the pinna e.g.
— hyperkeratosis
— Keloid
— Basal cell Ca.

b. Middle ear :

— Stapedectomy (Argon Laser).

c. Inner ear :

— Acoustic neuroma
— Meningioma.

* Pulsatile otorrhea is seen in ASOM.
* Eustachian tube is also known as pharyngotympanic tube.
* To distinguish cochlear and postcochlear damage, test done is **Bekesy audiometry.**
* In middle ear, smallest space is hypotympanum.
* Inner ear is present in petrous temporal bone.
* Semicircular canal is stimulated by linear acceleration.
* Threshold for Bone conduction is decreased and that for air conduction is increased in disease of middle ear.
* Ear infection causes throat infection through Eustachian tube.
* Promontory in middle ear medial wall is due to cochlear turn.
* **Type D tympanogram** is seen in acoustic neuroma.
* The purpose of vasodilators in the treatment of Meniere's disease is to combat the arteriolar spasm of strin vascularis.
* Treatment of antral polyp in a child is **Avulsion polypectomy.**

* Following is not seen in posterior rhinoscopy inferior meatus.
* Maxillary antrum is in relation of ethmoid bone.
* Maxillary sinus carcinoma may be caused by irradiation.
* In frontal mucocele, eyeball is shifted downwards outwards.
* **Blackening** of inferior turbinate is seen in diabetes mellitus.
* Hard nose is found in rhinoscleroma.
* In Tamil Nadu states is the incidence of rhinosporidiosis is **highest.**
* **Vidian neurectomy** has been used successfully in the treatment of vasomotor rhinitis.
* A patient with traumatic nasal deformity seen one month after the injury should have rhinoplasty as soon as possible.
* Indication of radiotherapy in nasopharyngeal angiofibroma is invasion of middle cranial fossa.
* Eustachian tube closure is done in endolymphatic sac decompression.
* **Waldayer's ring** as situated in naso & oropharynx.
* Laryngoscopic finding in laryngomalacia is indrawing of aryepiglottic folds.
* Best position for bronchoscopy trendelenberg.
* Abductors of vocal cord helps in respiration.
* During emergency tracheostomy, pressure on cricoid is applied to **stabilise the trachea**.
* The head should be maximally extended statements is true about the performing while a tracheostomy.
* Vocal cord paralysis on the left side in an elderly person is commonly with bronchogenic carcinoma.
* Stridor in a child without fever is due to foreign body.
* Dysphagia for fluids but not solids is seen in Achalasia cardia.
* Pulsion type of diverticulum is commons in the oesophagus.
* Treatment of a patient with Ca esophagus with malignant tracheal fistula is palliative surgery (Bypass).
* Submucous fibrosis is a premalignant condition.

* Inferior thyroid artery structures is a close anatomic relation of the recurrent laryngeal nerve.
* Foreign body aspiration is most common in Ant. apical segment.
* Unilateral (side of) neck pain in the upper 1/3 below the angle of mandible is due to malignancy throat.
* **Bezold's triad** is characteristic of Otosclerosis.
* **Jackson's safety triangle** is used for tracheostomy.
* The point above the inner canthus of the eye which is tender in acute frontal sinusitis is **McEwen's point.**
* The types of asthmas, another names of Laryngismus stridulus are **Kepp's, Millar's** and **Wickmann's.**
* A part of anterior ligament fastening the malleus to the wall of the tympanum is **Meckel's band.**
* Waldeyer's tonsillar ring is also called **Bickel's ring.**
* A point 1.25 inches above and 1.25 inches behind middle ext. auditory meatus, the proper spot to apply the trephine in abscess of the temporosphenoid lobe is **Baker's point.**
* Recessus superior membrane tympanical is **Prussak's.**
* Frog's nose is due to B/L ethmoidal polyp.
* Thyroid cartilage begins to ossify about 5 years before cricoid cartilage.
* Submentovertical view is best to show Ethmoid sinus.
* Congenital deafness due to partial aplasia of saccule and cochlear duct is **Scheibe's deafness.**
* Limbus fossa ovalis is also called **Vieussens ring.**
* Waldeyer's tonsillar ring is also called **Bickel ring.**
* Closure of the eye as a result of tactile or thermal stimulation of the deepest part of the external auditory meatus and tympanum is **Kehrer's reflex**.
* A point where the greater palatine nerve emerges from the greater palatine foramen is **Meglin point**.
* A point 1.25 inches above and 1.25 inches behind the middle ext. auditory meatus, the proper spot to apply the trephine abscess on the temporosphenoid lobe is **Barker's point.**

* A transient outpouching of the embryonic pharynx rostrad of the oropharyngeal membrane and caudal to Rathke's pouch is **Seassel's pouch.**
* Incisure cartilaginis meatus acoustic is **Santorini fissure.**
* Congenital deafness due to total lack of development of inner ear is **Michel deafness.**
* Fluid-filled spaces in the organ of Corti between the outer hair cells communicating with inner tunnel through the spaces between the pillar cells are **Nuel's sound.**
* Sound that is produced by a mixture of all frequencies of mechanical vibration perceptible as sound is **White sound.**
* Picking of the nose regarded as an early sign of cerebrospinal meningitis is **Lafora's sign.**
* A depressed area in the recessus epitympanicus below Prussak's space is **Kretschmann's space.**
* **Forschheimer's spots** seen on soft palate in rubella are Red bluish coloured.
* Cavitas trigeminalis is **Meckel's space.**
* Involuntary movements of the ears produced by auditory stimulation is **Preyer's reflex.**
* The space within the membranous labyrinth is **Cotunnius space.**
* Cochleopalpebral reflex is also called **Gault's reflex**.
* Sounds that originate within the ear such as tinnitus is **Entotic.**
* Tympanic membrane is concave into the outer ear canal, and is elliptical, 1.0 cm high and 0.9 cm wide respectively.
* There is a 20 fold increase in the force transmission of sound waves due to area discrepancies between the footplate of the stapes and the tympanic membrane.
* **Hallpike test** is for vestibular function.
* Mucous glands in the mucosa of the esophagus just above the cardia are **Cobelli's glands.**
* A space containing connective tissue between the vertebral column and the pharynx and esophagus is **Henke space.**
* Lymph nodes situated over the facial artery are **Stahr glands.**

* The space within the membranous labyrinth is **Cotunnius space**.
* Tubular mucous glands of the tongue are **Weber's.**
* **Nuel spaces** are found in organ of corti.
* **Wynn method** is used to repair cleft lip.
* Vertigo induced by high-intensity sounds in patients with circumscribed labyrinthitis is **Tullio phenomenon.**
* Closure of the eye as a result of tactile or thermal stimulation of the deepest part of the external auditory meatus and tympanum is **Kehrer's and Kisch's reflex.**
* Atresia of inner ear may be seen in the Turner's syndrome, trisomy and congenital rubella syndrome except Klinefelter's syndrome.
* Unilateral congestion of the ear upon stimulation of the distal end of the divided great auricular nerve is Snellen's reflex.
* Rhabdomyosarcoma is **most often** seen in orbit.
* Excessive salivation due to irritation of esophagus (esophagosalivary) is Roger reflex.
* After acoustic neuroma, second commonest CPA tumor is meningioma.
* Involuntary movements of the ears produces by the auditory stimulation is **Preyer reflex.**
* Stimulation of the semicircular canal causes nystagmus in place of that canal **Flouren's law**.
* **De Salle nasal lines** extend from the ala nasi in a semi circle around the mouth.
* A prone position employed after intubation so that the patient may swallow without danger of fluid entering the tube is **Casselberry position.**
* The making of rhythmic traction movements on the tongue in order to stimulate the respiratory centre in asphyxiation is Laborde method.
* In otitis media, the lateral sinus and cerebellum are liable to involvement in mastoid disease and the cerebrum may be attacked when the roof of the tympanum becomes çarious. This is **Fajan's law**.

* An operation to correct a flat nasal tip with short columella by using bilateral flaps of skin elevated in the hoor of the nostrils is **Dickinson method.**
* **Sluder method** is used to remove tonsils.
* In progressive organic diseases of the motor laryngeal nerves, the abductors of the vocal cords are the first, and occasionally the only muscles affected. This is **Semon Rosenbach law**.
* A method of examination of hypopharynx, with the cricoid cartilage drawn forward is **Eicken method.**
* Inspection of the larynx without a laryngoscope by having the patient incline his head far back and depressing the tongue is **Kirstein method.**
* **Vallecular narrowing** is seen in thyroglossal cyst.
* Serous secreting glands in the posterior part of the tongue near the valate papillae are **Ebner glands.**
* Reinke's edema of vocal cords may be seen in **Myxoedema.**
* Guerin fracture is Le Forte fracture type 1.
* Lymph nodes on the conold ligament at the upper border of the isthmus of the thyroid are **Poirier's glands.**
* Sluder's neuralgia originates from middle turbinate.
* Test which depends on the fact that to the normal man, the sound of his own voice is necessary for proper regulation of its tone and loudness is **Lombard test.**
* Glandulae thyroidae accessoriae or accessory thyroid glands are also called *Sandstrom's glands.*
* Anaesthesia of the tympanic membrane in otosclerosis is **Itard-Cholewa sign.**
* Pearly masses of epithelial cells near the surface of the gum of the infant are **Serres glands.**
* Becker's, Rosen's and Converse's operations are **Otoplasty operations.**
* Nose of divided into **5 areas** by Cottle.
* 'Squashed' nose most commonly results due to **Natal trauma.**
* Woodman operation is **External arytenoidectomy.**
* Refsum's, Leopard and Townes syndromes cause deafness.

# ANATOMY OF THE EAR

## DEVELOPMENT OF THE EAR

| *Ectoderm* | *Mesoderm* | *Endoderm* |
|---|---|---|
| External ear<br>auricle, external acoustic meatus, skin, glands | Middle ear<br>Upper ear<br>Ossicles and mastoid | Middle ear<br>lower half |
| Tympanic membrane<br>outer layer | Tympanic membrane<br>middle layer | Tympanic membrane<br>inner layer |
| Membranous labyrinth<br>Organ of Corti, utricle, saccule semicircular canals | Bony labyrinth<br>petrous temporal bone. | Auditory (Eustachian) tube. |

## EMBRYONIC TIME TABLE

| *Time in fetal weeks* | *Branchial apparatus external and middle ear* | *Otocyst membranous labyrinth* |
|---|---|---|
| 3 | First pharyngeal pouch | Otic placode |
| 4 | Primitive meatus | Otocyst |
| 6 | Hillocks | Endolymphatic sac and duct, Semicircular canals and cochlea |
| 8 | Solid epithelial core from primitive meatus towards tympanum | Cartilaginous otocyst |
| 12 | Hillocks fuse<br>Ossicles differentiating<br>Tympanic ring ossifies | Organ of Corti |

## EMBRYONIC TIME TABLE (Contd...)

| *Time in fetal weeks* | *Branchial apparatus external and middle ear* | *Otocyst membranous labyrinth* |
|---|---|---|
| 16 | Ossicles, fully formed in cartilage, begin to ossify | Fistula ante — fenestra appears<br>Ossification labyrinthine capsule begins |
| 23 | Pneumatization upper half tympanum and epitympanum<br>Antrum appears | Ossification labyrinthine<br>Capsule nearly complete |
| 28 | Solid epithelial, meatal core cannalizes | |
| 35 | Pneumatization of cells begins around antrum | |
| Birth | Pneumatization accelerates<br>Mastoid process appears | |
| Puberty | Osseus meatus complete, Pneumatization complete except for petrous | |

# PHYSIOLOGY OF HEARING

## TUNING FORK TESTS ANALYSIS

| | | *Rinne* | *Weber* | *ABC* |
|---|---|---|---|---|
| A. | Normal hearing ear | Positive | Central | Normal |
| B. | Conductive loss : | | | |
| | i) Right ear | Rt. ear-negative<br>Lt. ear-positive | Lateralised to right | Normal |
| | ii) Left ear | Rt. ear-positive<br>Lt. ear-negative | Lateralised to left | Normal |
| | iii) Bilateral | Both ear-negative | Lateralised to deafer side or no lateralisation, if equally deaf | Normal |
| C. | Sensorineural loss : | | | |
| | i) Right ear | Rt. ear-positive (low) | Lateralised to left | Rt. reduced. |
| | ii) Left ear | Rt. ear-positive<br><br>Lt. ear-positive (low) | Lateralised to right | Lt. reduced |
| | iii) Bilateral | Both ear-positive (low) | Lateralised to better ear or central, if equally deaf | Reduced-both |

## AUDIOLOGICAL TESTS

1. ***Pure Tone Audiometry :***

This is still by far the *commonest form* of audiometry performed. Air conduction and bone conduction hearing are tested by pure tone through an audiometer at octave steps i.e 125, 250, 500, 1000, 2000, 4000 and 8000 Hz. The intensity of sound is increased or decreased for each above frequency from 0 dB to 100 dB. The threshold of hearing at each frequency in A.C. and B.C. is plotted on a graph called audiogram. The frequency range between 500 and 3000 is more important in clinical practice.

*Applied importance :*

a) Diagnosis of conductive deafnes with air-borne (A-B) gap.

b) Diagnosis of sensori-neural deafness.

c) Diagnosis and confirmation of clinical otosclerosis. (A-B gap with Corhart's notch at 2000 in BC).

d) Diagnosis of **"acoustic trauma"**— sudden dip at 4000 of both BC & AC tracing.

2. ***Speech Audiometry :***

Is performed to measure the intelligibility of the spoken words in patients being tested. Recorded test words are played via head-phone at various sound pressure.

a) *Speech reception threshold :* The level at which the subject can repeat correctly 50% of spondee words.

b) *Speech discrimination test :* Phonetically balanced words are used to find the percentage intelligibility.

Applied Importance :

i) In conductive deafness or normal hearing : 95 to 100% speech discrimination score.

ii) In retro-cochlear sensori-neural deafness : score is low.

iii) In cochlear deafness : speech discrimination is better.

3. **Bekesy audiometry :**

This is a self-recording type of audiometry in which patient depresses or releases a button according to whether. He hears or ceases to hear the test tone and audiometric tracings are prepared.

*Applied Importance :*

i) Type I tracing is normal.

ii) Type II tracing suggests cochlear lesion.

iii) Type III & IV suggest retro-cochlear lesion.

iv) Type V suggests malingeering.

4. ***Tests for recruitment :***

a) Alternate Binaural Loudness Balance test (ABLB.) : This is also called ***Fowler's test.*** A tone is played alternately into normal and deaf ear above threshold and intensity is gradually increased until the sound is heard equally in both ear. The graph is called *laddergram.*

In negative recruitment angular orientation of the ladder remains regular. In positive recruitment, the ladder steps return to horizontal i.e. at higher intensity the sound is heard equally by deaf and normal ear.

Applied importance :

In a normal ear and conductive deafness the test is negative, but in cochlear deafness the test is positive.

b) ***Short Increment Sensitivity Index (SISI) Test :***

This test records the ability of the ear to recognise increase of 1 dB in the intensity of pure tone at 20 dB above threshold every 5 sec. The cycle occurs 20 times.

5. ***Threshold tone decay :***

A continuous tone is presented 5 dB above threshold in 500 and 2000 Hz. The result is expressed as the number of decibels by which intensity has to be increased in order to make the tone remain audible for 60 seconds.

If decay of 30 dB or more, retrocochlear lesion (acoustic neuroma) is almost certainly present.

6. ***Impedance audiometry :***

This valuable test provides a quick objective resistance measurement of state of tympanic membrane and middle ear and their compliance to sound pressure transmission.

*Tympanogram* is the graphic representation of the relative compliance and impedance of the tympanooccicular system with air-pressure changes.

*Applied importance :* 4 classical tracings are obtained :

Type A : Normal tympanogram. In otosclerosis graph is normal or compliance is slightly lower than normal.

Type B : Flat or dome shaped curve as in secretory otitis media.

Type C : Maximum compliance at negative pressure as in eustachian tube dysfunction.

Type D : Increased compliance at normal pressure as in ossicular chain disruption.

***Stapedial reflex***

Impedance audiometry can also be used to elicit stapedial reflex with sound of 70-95 dB above threshold. It is a *objective test* for :

i) Rough estimation of hearing ability.

ii) Detection of non-organ hearing loss (Malingeerers)

iii) Demonstration of recruitment.

iv) Localisation of lesion of the facial nerve.

v) Assessment of hearing of neonates and children.

This type of audiometry is becoming more and more popular due to its valuable guidance in diagnosis of various otological problems.

7. **Evoked Response Audiometry (E.R.A.)** : is the most recent advancement in audiology which is more objective in diagnosis of cochlear and retro-cochlear lesions.

*There are three main types :*

a) *Electro-Cochleography (E. coch. G) :* Records electrical activity generated in cochlea.

b) *Brain-stem audiometry (B.S.R.A) :* Records electrical response in cochlear nuclei and its central connections in brain-stem.

c) *Cortical evoked response audiometry (C.E.R.A) :* Electrical activity occurring in the vertex.

*Applied importance :*

1. Helps to detect retro-cochlear lesion.
2. Helpful in pediatric audiometry.
3. Diagnosis non-organic hearing-loss
4. Medico-legal aspects.

## HEARING-AIDS (AIDS TO HEARING)

When deafness is handicap to hear normal conversation and speech, then some form of artificial aid is necessary.

***Artificial hearing aids can be divided into :-***

A. *Non-electrical :* These are seldom used now-a-days. These are in the form of speaking tubes, ear trumpets, auricles and resonators amplifying about 15 dB—20 dB (gain).

B. *Electrical :* Modern electrical hearing-aid is a compact electronic device to amplify sound. It consists of :

   i) *Microphone :* Collects sound energy and converts it into electrical response.

   ii) *Amplifier :* Amplifies the sound.

   iii) *Receiver :* Built in ear-piece

   iv) *Power supply :* Consists of small battery.

***The basic varieties :***

a) Insert-type model.

b) Post-auricular model

c) Cosmetic models in Eye-glass frame, Ear-ring etc.

***Uses :***

1. *In conductive deafness* — Where operative procedure is unlikely to help or patient is unwilling to undergo operation.
2. *In sensori-neural deafness*—Helpful in some cases.
3. *Auditory training of deaf child*—Often binaural aid is used.

## NYSTAGMUS

### SPONTANEOUS NYSTAGMUS :

a) *First degree :* Nystagmus is produced only when patient looks in the direction of quick component.

b) *Second degree :* When produced by looking straight ahead.

c) *Third degree :* When produced by looking in the direction of slow component.

**INDUCED NYSTAGMUS :** Produced by rotational thermal or visual stimulation. Valuable information is obtained about vestibular system by utilising these stimuli and examining the nystagmus.

**COMMONLY USED TESTS ARE :**

1. ***Galvanic stimulation :*** Is of limited value.
2. ***Barany's rotation test :*** Post-rotatory nystagmus is measured.
3. ***Caloric test :*** Fitzgerald & hallpike technique.

   Patient lies supine with head flexed 30° forward to make the lateral semi-circular canal vertical. If water at 30°C (i.e. 7°C below and above normal temperature) is run in the external canal of each ear under standard condition, nystagmus is produced in a normal person with healthy labyrinth. The period of nystagmus is recorded on a calorigram. Application of a 20 + diopter lens (Frenzel glass) will prevent fixation or inhibition which can obscure the test. Normally the nystagmus lasts for about 2 to 3 mt. from the beginning of the stimulation.

   *Applied importance :*

   i) *Canal paresis :* Is present, if the duration of nystagmus is reduced for both hot and cold. This signifies peripheral vestibular lesion.

   ii) *Directional preponderance :* Means that bithermal testing yields a greater response to one direction than the other. This may be due to peripheral or central vestibular lesion.

4. *Cold-air test by Dundas-Grant method :* Is performed in a perforated ear drum.
5. *Cold caloric test with ice cold water* (**Obrak's test**) **:** Gives a rough guide of vestibular function.
6. *Fistulest :* A fistula in bony wall of the lateral semicircular canal may result from erosion by middle ear pathology (cholesteatoma) such as in chronic suppurative otitis media. Compression of air in the external canal will produce stimulation of lateral semicircular canal fluid through the fistula. Test is done by pressing the tragus and alternately releasing it or by compression by Siegle's speculum. Positive test is evident by presence of vertigo and nystagmus.

*Applied importance :*

1. *Positive fistula test :* Signifies presence of fistulous communication between middle ear and labyrinth.
2. *Negative fistula test :*
   a) Usually indicates absence of any fistula on the lateral semicir-cular canal.
   b) This is possible in a case of fistula, if the labyrinth is dead due to disease process (previous labyrinthitis).

*Surgical importance :*

Presence of positive fistula test is an important indication for early exploration of the mastoid.

7. ***Romberg's test :*** This is a useful test. Patient stands with eyes closed and feet together. Direction of swaying or falling is noted.

   *Applied importance :*

   Patient tends to fall to the side of peripheral lesion.

8. ***Electro-nystagmography :***Is the most modern and useful in the evaluation of vestibular disorder in which eye movements are graphically recorded. By placing electrodes at outer canthus of each eye and frontal region potential difference is picked up between cornea and retina and eye movements can be recorded.

*Applied importance :*

a) Shows spontaneous nystagmus.
b) Shows peripheral or central lesion.
c) Graphically records : No visual assessment as in caloric test.

9. ***Optokinetic nystagmus :***White drum with vertical black stripes is rotated in front of patient in both direction and the nystagmus is recorded.

   *Applied importance :*

   Asymmetry of response suggests central lesion.

# DISEASES OF THE EAR

## CAUSES OF EARACHE

| *Local causes* | *Referred causes* |
|---|---|
| 1. Furuncle of the ext. ear | 1. Dental causes : impacted wisdom tooth, caries, tooth apical, tooth abscess, gingivitis etc. |
| 2. Otitis externa. | 2. Tongue lesions : ulcer, glositis, malignancy etc. |
| 3. Impacted cerumen. | 3. Tonsillar lesions : acute tonsillitis, peritonsillar abscess, malignancy etc. |
| 4. Animate and impacted F. B. ext. canal | 4. Ulcer and inflammation of floor of the mouth |
| 5. Herpetic lesions. | 5. Pharyngeal lesions : abscess, ulcer, F.B., malignancy etc. |
| 6. Myringitis and traumatic rupture of tymp. membrane | 6. Laryngeal lesions : abscess, ulcer, F.B, malignancy etc. |
| 7. Acute otitis media, acute salpingitis, etc. | 7. Nasopharyngeal lesions : nasopharyngitis, infected adenoid, nasopharyngeal malignancy etc. |
| 8. Unsafe type of chr. supp. otitis media with threatening, complication | 8. Temporo-mandibular arthritis. |
| 9. Barotraumatic otitis media, haemotympanum etc. | 9. Acute maxillary sinusitis, nasal and maxillary malignant growth etc. |
| 10. Malignant growth of ext. & middle ear. | 10. Cervical spinal lesions, neck lesions etc. |

## DIFFERENT TYPES OF PERFORATIONS OF THE EAR & THEIR SIGNIFICANCE

| | *Type* | *Site & characteristic* | *Site of Pathology* | *Significance* |
|---|---|---|---|---|
| 1. | Central | in the pars tensa with all round. It can be of various sizes and in different quadrant of pars tensa. | Tubo-tympanic | i. Signifies safe type of rim of tym. membrane C.S.O.M.<br>ii. Cholesteatoma uncommon<br>iii. Complication usually absent |
| 2. | Marginal | Usually in the post-sup. margin of pars tensa and bony annulus is exposed i.e. one margin is formed by bony annulus and other sides by pars tensa. | Attico-antral | i. Signifies unsafe type of C.S.O.M.<br>ii. Cholesteatoma formation usual<br>iii. Various intra and extra-cranial complications may occur which often result in fatalities. |
| 3. | Attic | In the pars flaccida | Attico-antral | Same as marginal |

## DIFFERENCE BETWEEN SAFE AND UNSAFE EAR DISEASE

| | | *Safe* | *Unsafe Ear* |
|---|---|---|---|
| 1. | Otorrhea | Profuse; mucoid or muco-pus; non-foetid. | Scanty, thick, purulent & foetid. |
| 2. | Bleeding or Blood stained discharge | Nil | Often. |
| 3. | Deafness | Conductive-slight to moderate | Conductive moderate to severe; sometimes mixed. |
| 4. | Symptoms of complications such as headache, vertigo, etc. | Not present | May be present in advanced case |
| 5. | Perforation | Central | Attic or marginal |
| 6. | Granulation or Aural Polyp | Uncommon | Common |
| 7. | Fistula test | Negative | May be positive |
| 8. | Pathology | Tubo-tympanic disease | Attico-antral |
| 9. | Cholesteatoma | Uncommon | Common |
| 10. | Radiology | Cellular or hypocellular no bone erosion | Sclerotic bone; evidence of bone erosion common |
| 11. | Complication | Usually absent | Common |

## CAUSES OF SUDDEN SENSORINEURAL HEARING LOSS

* Barotrauma
* Ear/head injury
* Infection : mumps, measles, meningitis
* Cochlear otosclerosis
* CNS disease
* Previous ear surgery
* Ototoxic drugs
* Acoustic neuroma
* Multiple sclerosis
* Psychogenic factors

## CSOM - DIFFERENTIAL DIAGNOSIS

| *Safe Ear* | *Unsafe Ear* |
|---|---|
| * Tubotympanic | * Attico-antral infection |
| * Ascending infection | * Descending infection |
| * Benign chronic otitis media | * Dangerous chronic otitis media |
| * Anterior or Central perforation | * Attic or marginal perforation |
| * Profuse, mucoid odourless pus | * Scanty, thick, fetid odour pus |
| * Granulations—uncommon | * Granulations—common |
| * Pale & oedematous polypus | * Hyperaeimic & fleshy polypus |
| * Slight to moderate conductive deafness | * Moderate to severe conductive mixed deafness |
| * Average normal mastoid cell X-size & number on X-ray | * Absence of mastoid air cells on ray |
| * Cholesteatoma—very uncommon | * Cholesteatoma—very common |
| * Good prognosis | * Bad prognosis |

# DIFFERENCE BETWEEN CONDUCTIVE AND SENSORI-NEURAL DEAFNESS

| | *Conductive deafness* | *Perceptive deafness or sensori- neural deafness* |
|---|---|---|
| 1. Congenital | Less common | More common |
| 2. History | | |
| a) Onset | Mainly progressive, sudden less often | Sudden as well as progressive |
| b) History of viral fever, exanthematous fevers | Nil | Common after measles, mumps etc. |
| c) History of head injury | Less common | More common |
| d) History of prolonged medication | Nil | Often present |
| e) History of Otorrhoea. | Often present | Nil |
| f) History of Vertigo | Occasional | More common |
| g) History of Noise and sound trauma. | Nil | May be present. |
| 3. Voice | Speaks in low tone. | Speaks in loud voice |
| 4. Noise intolerance | No | Yes |
| 5. Paracusis | May be present in otosclerosis | No |
| 6. Speech discrimination | Good | Poor |
| 7. Tuning fork tests | | |
| a) Rinne | Negative i.e. BC>AC | Positive (low) AC > BC |
| b) Weber | Lateralised to deaf ear | Lateralised to better ear |
| c) A.B.C. test | Normal | Shortened |
| 8. Audimetry | | |
| a) Pure tone | Confirms; good air-bone gap; low tone . loss common | Confirms; interwoven air and bone con duction; high tone loss |
| b) Speech | Good discrimination score. | Poor |
| c) Recruitment | Nil | Positive in cochlear deafness |

## DIFFERENCE BETWEEN CONDUCTIVE AND SENSORI-NEURAL DEAFNESS (Contd..)

| | *Conductive deafness* | *Perceptive deafness or sensori- neural deafness* |
|---|---|---|
| d) Tympanometry | Helps in secretory O.M. Ossicular. disruption etc | No |
| e) Tone decay | Not present | Present in retro-cochlear deafness. |
| f) Brain stem audiometry, cortical response audiometry | No | Helps in diagnosis in retrocochlear deafness. |

## TREATMENT OF CHOICE (EXTERNAL EAR)

**AURICLE**

* Minor degrees of bat ear —*No treatment*
* Very pronounced deformity of bat ear—*Corrective operation of pinnaplasty.*
* External auditory meatus atresia with severe impairment of inner ear function—*Operation does not improve hearing.*
* Haematoma of auricle (before coagulation of blood)—*Wide bore needle aspiration under aseptic precautions.*
* Haematoma of the auricle (long standing cases)—*Incision & evacuation of the clot* (Treatment of choice).
* Seroma of the auricle—*Same as treatment of haematoma.*
* Impetigo of auricle—*bathing with warm sterile saline + Neomycin cream.*
* Subperichondrial abscess—*Incision & Drainage.*
* Chondrodermatitis nodularis chronicis helicis—local excision (including a small wedge of the underlying cartilage).
* *Tophi—treat the underlying condition.*
* Symptomatic Dermoid cyst of preauricular fistula—*Excision.*
* Sebaceous cysts of auricle—*Excision.*

* Incisional cysts—
    * Small cysts—*Evacuated*
    * Large cysts—*Excision*
    * Recurrent cyst—*Total excision*
* Large warts & horns of auricle—*Excision*
* Squamous cell carcinoma of auricle—
    * Small lesions on Upper half—*Wedge incision with wide margin of healthy tissue.*
    * Large lesions on lower half—*Total excision of pinna.*
* Basal cell carcinoma —
    * Rodent ulcers of the pinna—*Excision together with a margin of healthy tissue.*
    * Very small superficial lesions—*radiotherapy.*
    * Advanced cases with infiltration of the underlying bone—*Wide excision & post-operative radiotherapy.*

---

## EXTERNAL AUDITORY MEATUS

---

* Acquired meatus atresia
    * Minor variety without symptoms—*No treatment.*
    * Severe variety or Total occlusion of deep meatus causing conductive deafness—*Surgical correction.*
* Contracture of meatal introitus (due to burns, lacerations) or stenosed meatus (after mastoid surgery)—*meatoplasty.*
* Impacted wax—*Dissolve wax with olive oil followed by syringing.*
* Impacted wax in special situations & in patients with past history of ear trouble—*Removal under direct vision* (using ring-ended probe, or blunt hook or aural dressing forceps).

**Foreign Bodies in the Ear :**

* Flies or insects—*Killed by instilling spirit into the external auditory meatus followed by syringing.*
* Maggots—*Application of chloroform water or vapour (to kill maggots) followed by syringing.*
* Vegetable foreign bodies—*Removal under direct vision with small forceps or blunt hook.*

---

* Large foreign bodies—*Removal under direct vision with small forceps or blunt hook.*
* Foreign body impacted in deep meatus—*Renoved by opening the meatus through post auricular incision.*

**Otitis externa**—*Removal of all debris and discharge from the ear canal.*

**Furunculosis**—*Local & general measures*

* Local treatment—*Local heat application, meatal packs (10% ichthammol glycerin) & cleansing.*
* General treatment—*Flucloxacillin, 5-day course.*
* Boil pointing on the skin—*Incision.*
* Recurrent cases—*Chlorhexidine or neomycin cream local application for several days.*
* Diffuse otitis externa—*thorough & gently irrigation of meatus with isotonic saline & dry mopping + Gentamycin ear drops.*

  * Chronic stage—meticulous toilet of the meatus + antiseptic & hydrocortisone cream or ear drops.
* Otomycosis—Through cleansing of the meatus & dry mopping + Nystatin, clotrimazole or econazole lotion (Amphotericin-B for candida infections) *for 3 to 4 weeks.*
* Seborrhoeic dermatitis—*Scalp condition to be controlled by regular selenium sulphide shampoos + meatal cleaning + local ointment (salicyclic acid + precipitated sulphur + petroleum jelly).*
* Dermatitis of the auricle—*Anti-inflammatory antiallergic steroids + Antibacterial agents.*

**Otitis externa haemorrhagic** (Bullous myringitis)—*Analgesics* (Antibiotics have no influence & incision of bleb is of no value).

**Malignant Otitis externa**—Removal of granulation tissue + Excision of necrotic tissue from meatus of infection — wide surgical excision of all infected tissue & bone).

**Herpes zoter Otiticus (Ramsay Hunt's syndrome)**—

* Herpes auricularis—*No curative treatment, protection of vesicles by antipruritics (hydrocortisone acetate) & Pain is releived by aspirin.*

* Herpes auricularis with facial pasly—*Local treatment as aboe + Total surgical decompression of geniculate ganglion.*
* Herpes auricularis with facial palsy & auditory symptoms—Bed rest with labyrinthine sedations (Promethazine) + *prednisolone* + *Local treatment* (as above).
* Basal cell carcinoma—*Radical excision combined with post-operative radiotherapy.*
* Adenocarcinoma—*Radical surgery combined with postoperative radiotherapy.*

## EXTERNAL EAR OPERATIONS

***Pinnaplasty***—Operative procedure for correction of auricular protrusion.

*Indication*—bat ear (congenital failure of formation of antihelix).

*Complications :*

* Perichondritis
* Cauliflower ear (haematoma auris)

***Meatoplasty***—Operative procedure for improvement of shape & size of external auditory canal.

*Indications :*

* Chonchal cartilage congenital deformity (with or without meatal atresia)
* Acquired meatal atresia.

*Contraindications*

* Perichondritis
* Restenosis (post-operative)

***Myringotomy*** —Incision of tympanic membrane

*Indications for Posterior myringotomy:*

* Tense middle ear pus
* Non-purulent middle ear effusion (secretory otitis media)

*Complications :*

* Incudostapedial joint or ossicles injury
* Jugular bulb (floor of middle ear) injury
* Chorda tympani injury

*Indications for Anterior Myringotomy incision.*

* Grommet tube insertion
* Tympanic effusion aspiration
* *Treatment contraindications for tympanic membrane rupture or injury*
  * Do not clean out the eat
  * Do not remove the clot
  * Do not wet the ear
  * Do not put in drops
  * Do not syringe
  * Do not interfere
* Syringing should not be used if there is a past history of ear trouble.
* Forceps should never be used while attempting removal of smooth round foreign bodies from external auditory meatus.
* The essential defect of bat ear is failure of formation of the antihelical convexity
* Squamous carcinoma occurring on the upper half of the auricle carry a fat better prognosis than those in the lower half.

## TREATMENT OF CHOICE (MIDDLE EAR)

### ACUTE OTITIS MEDIA :

* Acute otitis media in infancy—*Full course of antibiotics* (SOS—if persistent of pain if pain increases *Myringotomy of swab for C/S).*
* Acute catarrhal otitis media in childhood—*Nasal decongestants to re-open. Eustachian tube* (SOS—*Politzerization, myringotomy).*
* Recurring attacks of catarrhal otitis media with succeeding head colds & persisting slight hearing loss with indrawn eardrums in children—*Adenoidectomy (if enlarge) or treatment for allergic rhinitis.*
* Acute suppurative otitis media in childhood—
  * Without discharge—Amoxycillin or Ampicillin i.m for 2 days followed by oral for 1 wk.
  * With discharge—Swab for c/s+ appropriate antibiotics + Nasal decongestants + Analgesics.

* Recurrent ASOM + Adenoiditis or Adenotonsillitis—Surgical removal of Adenoids & tonsils.
* Frequency of ear infection in childhood is reduced by—*Insertion of grommets.*
* Seasonal otitis media in childhood—*Prophylactic antibiotics* (half the standard dose over the period of risk).
* Eustachian tube dysfunction—*auto infection, elimination of infection in nose, sinuses & postnasal space, local or systemic decongestants.* (SOS—Posterior end of inferior turbinate impinges Eustachian tube—*Removal of malberry enlargement).*
* Abnormal patency of Eustachian tube :
  * Symptomatic relief—*Insertion of grommet.*
  * Destressing symptoms—*Teflon paste injecting into anterior Eustachian cushion.*
* Acute catarrhal otitis media —*Expectant treatment includes Nasal decongestants (axymetazoline). Eustachian tube inflation (Valsalvaauto-inflation, Politzerization or Eustachian tube catheterization).*
* Acute middle-ear effusion—*Treatment same as catarrhal otitis media* (If fluid & deafness persists—*Myringotomy).*

**Secretory otitis Media**

* Established case of secretory otitis media (Glue ear)—*Myringotomy & aspiration of fluid under GA.*
* Treatment of retraction pocket (with mobile lining) of secretory otitis media—*Excision of pocket + Insertion of grommet + removal of adenoids.*

## CHRONIC OTITIS MEDIA

* Chronic middle-ear effusion—*Myringotomy + grommet insertion (even in presence of postnasal tumours).*
* Chronic middle-ear effusion with collapsed or atrophic drum—*Grommets insertion anteriorly* (If atelectasis is long standing—*Hearing aid).*

* Persistence of chronic middle-ear effusion after this grommets have come out—*Long term ventilation tubes* (T-tube or titanium tubes).
* Tubotymponic otitis media—*Eliminating upper respiratory tract infection (Removal of tonsils, adenoids, or treatment of sinusitis)* + *local ear treatment by cleaning & antibiotic cream* (gentamycin + hydrocortisone).
* Tubotympanic otitis media with recurring discharge or deafness—Closure of perforation by myringoplasty).

**SAFE C.S.O.M : TUBOTYMPANIC DISEASE :**

* Active : Chronic or recently activated discharge from tubotympanic portion of the middle ear —*Local medical treatment & removal of polypus* + weekly observation.
* If persistent activity—Investigate & treat :
  * Upper respiratory tract—Permanent precautions
  * Mastoid air cells—Simple mastoidectomy
* Quiescent : An ear that has been recently discharging but has become dry—Monthly observation for 6 months (if persistent perforation—Permanent precautions or Myringoplasty).
* Inactive : If there has been no discharge from the middle ear for 6 months - with existence of tympanic membrane perforation—*Myringoplasty.* (If reperforation—*Remyringoplasty or permanent precaution).*

**UNSAFE C.S.O.M. : Attico-antral disease :**

* *Active disease :*
  * With cholesteatoma is visible or suspected on radiological or other grounds—*Tympanoplasty or Radical mastoidectomy.*
  * *With aural polypus :* An aural polyp extruded through or occluding perforation—*Removal of polypus.*
  * With granulations : granuloma may impede drainage & constitute irreversibly diseased tissue that cannot respond to aural toilet or topical medication— i) Small granulations — reduced by repeated cauterization with a fused silver nitrate bead; ii) Larger granulations—removal with cup forceps.

  * Cholesteatoma, polyp & granulation-free ear : Discharging pus along through well defined posterior or attic perforation—Local medical treatment, *twice weekly observation.*
  * Failed medical treatment—*tympanoplasty or Radical mastoidectomy.*
  * Doubtful assessment—*Examination under anaesthesia & S.O.S.* —Surgery.
  * Complicated : Spread of disease into adjacent areas i.e. Facial nerve palsy, labyrinthitis & intracranial extension—*Radical mastoidectomy.*

* ***Quiscent :*** An ear that has been discharging from an unsafe area but which has recently become dry, either spontaneously or under the influence of conservative medical treatment—*Monthly observation* (if persistent perforation—*Permanent precautions).*
* ***Tuberculous otitis media***—General treatment—Intensive chemotherapy with antituberculous drugs + Local treatment of — aural toilet, insufflation of streptomycin powder & surgical excision of necrotic tissue.
* ***Syphilic otitis media***—General treatment—Specific antisyphilitic treatment + Local treatment—keep the ear clean, reduce secondary infection & maintain free drainage.
* ***Adhesive otitis media*** —Exploratory tympanotomy to discover the exact nature of pathology & by appropriate technique to restore mobility (if possible) + provision of hearing aid.

## OTOSCLEROSIS

* Early stages—*Regular observation.*
* When operation is contraindicated or opposed by patient—Hearing aid & lip-reading tution + Rehabilitation at work.
* Choice of treatment in favourable cases—*Stapedectomy with total or partial removal of the footplate.*

## TUMOURS OF MIDDLE EAR

***Squamous cell carcinoma of middle ear & mastoid :***

* Growth believed to be confined to middle ear and mastoid. No palpable enlargement of regional lymph glands — *Subtotal excision of temporal bone (at least radical mastoidectomy) to include facial nerve, if involved, followed by radiotherapy.*
* Growth suspected of extension beyond middle ear and mastoid—
* Into petrous (vertigo, sensorineural deafness) but not into cranial cavity (no nerve palsy except VIIth and VIIIth; no CNS signs)— Subtotal excision of temporal bone with readiness to follow disease to the limits of operability, followed by radiotherapy.
* Into cranial cavity (nerve palsies and other CNS signs)— Radiotherapy only.
* Into parotid gland or temporomandibular joint—Careful decision as to operability. If in doubt, radiotherapy only.
* Into cartilaginous portion of auditory tube (growth visible at pharyngeal opening)—*Radiotherapy only.*
* Growth, regardless of apparent local extent, associated with secondary deposit in regional lymph glands —*Subtotal excision of temporal bone, radiotherapy, or combined.*
* Growth associated with severe uncontrolable intractable pain following radiotherapy only, especially applicable above, without obvious intracranial extension—*Total excision of temporal bone* (or subtotal if object of major growth elimination would seem achieved thereby).

***Glomus jugulare tumour :***

* *Group I Aural symptoms only ± VIIth-nerve palsy*
  * Symptoms sight, tumour observed through intact membrane—*Tympanotomy* (myringomeatal flap) and *biopsy excision bleeding controlled by coagulation diarthermy, gelfoam, and packing; Prolonged regular observation.* (These cases may remain in status quo for many years). *Any sign of recurrence may be regarded as indication for radiotherapy.*

* Symptoms severe, i.e. VIIth-nerve palsy, membrane breached by glomus (polyp)—*Biopsy: radical mastoidectomy (or combined approach tympanoplasty with posterior tympanotomy) to expose extent of tumour mass as far as possible without trauma.*
* Group II, III and IV, with neurological involvement — *Radiotherapy*

## MIDDLE EAR OPERATIONS (SIMPLE OR CONSERVATIVE)

***Anterior tympanotomy :***

—Exposure of tympanic cavity

* *Indications :*
    * *Diagnosis*—Exploratory tympanotomy
    * *High viscosity effusion*—drainage
    * *Complications*—Otitis media

***Cortical (Simple or conservative) mastoidectomy (Swartze operation)***

— (Removal of mastoid air cells w/o disturbing middle ear contents)

* *Indications :*
    * Acute empyema of mastoid
    * Persistent profuse otorrhoea
    * Recurrent otitis media
    * Marked mastoiditis
* *Complications :*
    * Facial nerve injury
    * Dislocation of incus
    * Penetration of lateral venous sinus
    * Penetration of middle fossa dura
    * Postoperative haematoma
    * Postoperative pus reaccumulation
    * Cochlear injury

* ***Radical mastoidectomy :*** (Classical operation) : Removal of disease process in tympanic cavity & mastoid antrum by forming single bony cavity which communicates freely with external meatus (Structures removed—tympanic membrane, malleus, incus, chorda tympani & mucoperiosteal lining).
* *Indications :*
    * Unsafe CSOM
    * Cholesteatoma
    * Complications of CSOM
* Maligant disease of middle ear
* As an exposure for surgical treatment of —
    * Radical (bony) labyrinthectomy (suppurative labyrinthitis).
    * Drainage of petrous apex (apical petrositis).
    * Grafting or decompression of facial nerve.
    * Drainage of extradural abscess.
* *Complications :*
    * Facial nerve palsy
    * Suppurative labyrinthitis
    * Severe conductive deafness
    * Unhealed cavity

***Modified radical mastoidectomy*** (Attico-antrostomy)—Operative procedure for clearance of disease processes localized to the epithympanum (attic) & mastoid antrum.

* *Modified radical mastoidectomy*—Removal from without inwards.
* *Attic-antrostomy*—Removal of bone from within outwards (starting from tympanic cavity).
* *Indications :*
    * Epidermoid cholesteatoma
    * Localised chronic otitis media
    * As a preliminary surgical procedure (for fenestration operation).
* *Complications :*
    * Disease recurrence
    * Facial nerve palsy
    * Unhealed cavity

**Combined approach mastoidectomy** (Intact-canal-wall mastoidectomy):

— Useful for exposure & clearance of disease from middle ear cleft by retaining postmeatal wall intact (as a preliminary to tympanoplasty).

* *Indications :*
  * Unsafe chronic otitis media
  * Cholesteatoma
* *Contraindications:*
  * Threatened or manifest complications of middle ear
  * Malignancy
* *Complications :*
  * Recurrence of infection of cholesteatoma.

***Tympanoplasty :***

* Operation for reconstruction of sound-conducting apparatus for middle ear.
* Consists repair of tympanic membrane (myringoplasty) & repair of ossicular chain (ossiculoplasty).
* *Indications :*
  * Loss of complete or part of tympanic membrane & ossicles due to
  * Destructive disease
  * Trauma
  * Surgical excision
* *Contraindications :*
  * Obstruction of auditory tube (unreliable)
  * Sensorineural deafness (with no-air-bone gap on audiometry)
* *Complications :*
  * Fascia graft sloughing
  * Bone or cartilage graft displacement
  * Worsening of hearing
  * Dead ear
  * Infection

***Stapedectomy :***

* For relief of conductive deafness due to stapedial ankylosis.
* Re-establishment of linkage between incus & oval window by interposing teflon or stainless-steel piston.
* Vein graft is used for protection of vestibule.
* *Indications :*
  * Otosclerosis
  * Adhesive otitis
* *Contraindications :*
  * Sepsis—active otitis media
  * Sensorineural deafness
  * Severe irremediable deafness
  * Previous stapedectomy in other ear
  * Tympanic membrane—perforation or badly scarred & adherent.
* *Contraindications :*
  * Cochlear function loss
  * Perilymph fistula
  * Postop. dislocation of link
  * Chronic vertigo (mild)
  * Facial nerve palsy
  * Infection—Acute labyrinthitis & meningitis

***Mobilization Operation :***

Mobilization of stapes for relief of conductive deafness due to stapedial ankylosis (flap of skin created from external meatus is used to cover the fenestra).

* *Indications :*
  * Otosclerosis
  * Adhesive otitis
* *Contraindications :*
  * Infection—active otitis media or externa
  * Sensorineural deafness
  * Tympanic membrane perforation
  * Old age

* *Complications :*
    * Postop. vertigo
    * Facial nerve palsy
    * Cochlear function loss
    * Chronic mastoid cavity infection

## OPERATIONS OF THE EAR

### Myringotomy

It is incision of the tympanic membrane and drainage of the middle ear

*Indications :*

1. Acute suppurative otitis media :
    a) Bulged tympanic membrane on the point of rupture.
    b) If severe earache persists in a child inspite of treatment and the child is restless and is having disturbed sleep.
    c) Inadequate drainage—small pulsating perforation.
    d) Acute otitis media with complication.
    e) Delayed resolution.
2. Secretory otitis media.
3. Baro-traumatic otitis media, if conservative treatment fails.
4. Unresolved otitis media.
5. Some cases of adhesive otitis media and atelectasis.

*Complications :*

a) Injury to the ossicles, commonly incus and incudo-stapedial joint.
b) Injury to the inner ear through the round window.
c) Injury of jugular bulb in the hypotympanum, if high up.
d) Endomeatal : In stapedectomy and tympanotomy.

## COCHLEAR IMPLANTS

Provide electrical stimulation of cochlea by sound waves in cases of total deafness

* Types include :
    * Single channel implant
    * Multi channel implant

* Useful in the totally deaf to provide auditory rhythm signal & can greatly aid lip reading.
* Discrimination for speech is still primitive.
* Cochlear implants are a useful addition of rehabilitation of the totally deaf.
* *Selection of patients include—*
    * Acquired deafness beyond the reach of hearing aid.
    * Absence of active CSOM
    * Well motivated patients without debilitating disease

---

## TREATMENT OF CHOICE (INNER EAR)

---

**Deafness in children**

* Bilateral meatal atresia —*Surgery.*
* *Congenital deafness—*
* Prophylactic treatment—*Avoidance of predisposing factors* (consanguinity, intermarriage of born deaf, exposure to ototoxic drugs & rubella during early pregnancy) : Estimation of parents Rhesus groups & desensitization of susceptible mothers. Screening tests between 7 & 9 months of age of all children.
* Therapeutic treatment—*Cochlear implants.*
* Educational treatment—*Auditory training : Lip reading, Sign language, Speech training & Family guidance.*
* Sensorineural deafness in both ears in children—*Continued guidance & help from people throughout the child's life* (No surgical management of this condition).
* As early as 8 months old—*hearing aids.*
* Education of child—*Radio aids + Lip reading.*
* Any deaf child—*Binaural hearing.*
* Less severely deaf child—*in-the ear or module-type aids.*
* Child with mixed type of deafness (35-45 dB loss)—*needs favourable positioning in class, understanding primary teacher & constant help from visiting teacher.*

---

* Unilateral deafness in children—*Child must always be placed with the good ear towards the teacher and child sits with the deaf ear next to the wall* (in the room).

**Meniere's disease**—Medical treatment

* Reassurance
* Antihistamine labyrinthine sedatives.
* Vasodilator drugs (Betahistine hydrochloride, nicotinic acid derivatives, naftidrofuryl & cyclandelate).
* Improvement of general physical & mental health.
* Fluid & salt restriction.
* Diuretics.
* Meniere's disease—during acute attack—Sedative & labyrinthine sedatives.
* Meniere's disease with vertiginous attacks are crippling & unrelieved by medical measures.
    * Decompression of endolymphatic sac or drainage of succus endolymphaticus by simple exposure or incision.
    * Vestibular neurectomy
    * Cervical sympathectomy
    * Stellate ganglionectomy
    * Endolymph-perilymph shunting operations.
    * Selective labyrinthine destruction with preservation of hearing by ultrasound.
* Viral labyrinthitis—Symptomatic treatment.
* Bacterial labyrinthitis—Treatment of the cause.
* Labyrinthitis secondary to meningitis—Treatment of meningitis + symptomatic treatment of vertigo.
* Labyrinthine trauma—Non operative —bed rest & labyrinthine sedatives.
* Perilymph fistula—Surgical repair of the fistula by covering with fat or fascia.
* Vertigo due to CNS neoplasms, posterior-inferior cerebellar artery thrombosis & vertebrobasilar ischaemia—Treat the underlying cause.

**Facial nerve palsy :**

* Bell's palsy—
    * Steroids in various forms (ACTH, prednisolone, cortisone)
    * Surgical decompression of nerve.
    * Total decompression from the internal auditory meatus to stylomastoid foramen.
* Tumours (Acoustic neuroma & parotid gland tumours) involving facial nerve—Removal of underlying tumour + Excision of affected portion of nerve + Interpositional nerve graft.
* Acute otitis media complicated by facial paralysis—Operative intervention & drainage through myringotomy incision.
* Facial paralysis complicating cholesteatoma with erosion of Fallopian canal—Exploration of mastoid.
* Hemifacial spasm—Posterior craniotomy & elevation of abnormal vascular loop away from the facial nerve.

## INNER EAR OPERATIONS

***Membranous labyrinthectomy :***

Removal of membranous portion of the lateral semicircular canal

*Indications :*

* Indicated in Meniere's disease, when—
    * Disease is unilateral.
    * Hearing in affected ear is substantially impaired.
    * Failed medical treatment.

*Complications :*

* Total loss of cochlear function in operated ear (always).
* Postoperative vomiting & vertigo (usual).
* Infection (rare).

**Bony labyrinthectomy** (radical-total labyrinthectomy)

exanteration of labyrinth at, or after, radical mastoidectomy.

*Indications :*

* Suppurative labyrinthitis (when spread of infection to intracranial cavity is threatened)
* Persisting vestibular symptoms after mastoid surgery).

*Complications :*

* Total loss of hearing in operated ear (always)
* Facial nerve palsy
* Cerebrospinal otorrhea
* Post. operative vomiting & vertigo
* Persistence of vertigo

*Ultrasound labyrinthectomy :*

— Ultrasound irradiation for functional destruction of the labyrinth and preservation of hearing.

* Meniere's disease
* Residual vertigo (after membranous or bony labyrinthectom).

*Complications :*

* Facial nerve palsy
* Sensorineural deafness

*Facial nerve decompression :*

— Relieving pressure affect on facial nerve in tympanic or mastoid course.

*Indications :*

* Bell's palsy (ischaemic oedema).
* Facial nerve injury (fracture or surgical trauma).
* Disease (otitis media or inflammatory oedema).

# ANATOMY OF THE NOSE

*Meatuses & Openings :*

* Spheno ethmoidal recess—Sphenoid sinus (Space above superior turbinate).
* Superior meatus—Posterior ethmoidal sinuses.
* Middle meatus—Anterior group of sinuses.
    * Frontal sinus
    * Anterior ethmoidal sinus
    * Maxillary sinus
* Inferior meatus—Nasolacrimal ducts
* Nasal septum is bony (posteriorly) & cartilagious (anteriorly).

*Arterial supply of Septum :*

* Main source —External carotid system—> Maxillary artery—> Sphenopalatine artery.
    * Inferior turbinate artery
    * Middle turbinate artery
    * Nasopalatine artery (2 branches)
* Lesser source —Internal carotid system—>Ophthalmic artery—>Anterior ethmoidal artery.
* *Other vessels :*
    * Greater palatine (Maxillary artery branch).
    * Superior labial artery (Facial artery branch).
    * Infraorbital & superior dental artery (maxillary & pharyngeal branches of maxillary artery).
    * Posterior ethmoidal (Ophthalmic artery branch).
    * Little's area or Kiesselbach's plexus is a highly vascularised area at the anteroinferior aspect of septum with the above vessels.

## PARANASAL SINUSES

***Maxillary Sinuses :***

- * Antrum of Highmore.
- * Adult has a capacity of 15 ml & size 35 mm height, 300 mm anteroposteriorly.
- * Maxillary sinus ostium (in the upper part of its medial wall opens into the hiatus semilunaris of middle meatus).
- * *Relations—*
  - * Apex — Malar process
  - * Base — Lower part of lateral wall of nose
  - * Roof — Floor of orbit
  - * Floor — Alveolar process of maxilla & roots of the second premolar & first two molar teeth.
  - * Medial wall — Lateral wall of nasal cavity
  - * Posterior wall — Anterior wall of pterygopalatine & infratemporal fossa
- * Maxillary sinus is lined with ciliated columnar epithelium.

***Frontal sinuses :***

- * Arise from anterior ethmoidal cells & rudimentary at birth.
- * Situated in the frontal bone above supra orbital margin & root of nose.
- * Frontonasal duct opens into middle meatus.
- * *Relations :*
  - * Anterior wall — outer table
  - * Posterior wall — inner table
  - * Floor — orbital roof
  - * Medial wall — inner frontal sinus septum

***Ethmoid sinuses :***

- * Present at birth & grows extremely slowly.
- * Anterior group drains into middle meatus & posterior group drains into superior meatus.

***Sphenoid Sinuses :***

* Present at birth & true growth occurs at puberty.
* Sphenoidal sinus ostium drains into sphenoethmoidal recess.

***Radiography best view of Sinuses :***

* Occipitomental view — Maxillary antrum
* Occipitofrontal view — Ethmoidal sinuses & Frontal sinuses
  (Straight-on view) —
* Lateral view — Sphenoid sinus (nasopharynx & adenoid demonstration)
* Submentovertical view — Ethmoids & Sphenoid sinuses
* Oblique views — Ethmoids
* Tomograms of sinuses — Assessment of sinusitis, sinus tumours & bone destruction
* Fluid level — Diagnostic of infection
* Fluid level with total opacification — Gross infection or huge polyp
* Orthopantomogram — Dental examination

**INVESTIGATION OF CHOICE**

* Dysphagia lusoria — Lipiodal swallow or arteriography & Bronchoscopy
* Laryngomalacia — Laryngoscopy (direct) & flexible fibrescopy.
* Subglottic stenosis — Direct laryngoscopy & bronchoscopy
* Laryngotracheal cleft — Barium swallow followed by direct laryngoscopy
* Laryngeal web — Direct or fibreoptic laryngoscope

# LITTLE'S AREA

It is an area situated in the antero-inferior part of the septum where several vessels supplying the nasal cavity have anastomosed. As this area is very vascular, slightest trauma may precipitate bleeding per nose. This area is liable to trauma by nose-picking as well as external trauma. This vascular plexus is called **Kiesselbach's plexus.** Vessels which anastomose here are :

a) Anterior ethmoidal artery—septal branch

b) Greater palatine artery—septal branch

c) Spheno-palatine artery—septal branch

d) Septal branch of the superior labial artery.

Greatest contribution is from spheno-palatine artery, which is often termed *"artery of epistaxis"* and then anterior ethmoidal.

Bleeding sometimes may be profuse due to spurting arterioles.

**Surgical importance :**

1. One of the commonest site of epistaxis.
2. Common site of trauma by picking and external trauma.
3. Site of vascular anastomosis
4. Angioma may occur at the site — "bleeding polyp of the septum."

# DISEASES OF THE NOSE

## DIFFERENTIAL DIAGNOSIS OF EPISTAXIS

A. ***Local causes***

1. *Congenital :* Telangiectasis of the nose (Osler-Rendu Syndrome).
2. *Traumatic :*
   a) Physical trauma : Blows, fracture nose, external trauma, picking etc.
   b) Operative ; :Following operations in the nose.
   c) Chemical trauma : Workers of chemical factories
   d) Thermal trauma : Excessive heat.
   e) Foreign body
3. *Inflammatory or infective :*

| | | | |
|---|---|---|---|
| a) | Acute | : | Acute rhinitis, sinusitis. |
| | Specific | : | Nasal diphtheria |
| b) | Chronic | : | Rhinitis, sinusitis |
| | Specific | : | Tuberculosis, Syphilis etc. |
| c) | Fungal | : | Rhinosporidiosis |
| | Non-specific | : | Atrophic rhinitis. |

4. *Neoplastic :*
   a) Benign : Haemangioma, angioma of septum, papilloma, nasopharyngeal fibroma.
   b) Malignant : Carcinoma of the nose, paranasal sinuses and naso-pharynx.
5. *Circulatory :* Back pressure from enlarged adenoids.
6. *Miscellaneous :* Malignant granuloma; Bleeding from Little's area (often spontaneous) and Idiopathic.
7. *Environmental :* Drying of nasal mucosa.

B. ***Systemic or general causes :***

1. *Congenital :* Haemophilia and other coagulating disorders.
2. *Traumatic :* Fracture of anterior cranial fossa.
3. *Inflammatory :* (a) Acute exanthematous fevers e.g. (measles, pox, etc.) ; Acute malaria, typhoid, flu etc. (b) Chronic debilitating diseases.
4. *Neoplastic :*
   a) Leukaemia, Hodgkin's disease
   b) Malignant : Lymphosarcoma.
5. *Blood dyscrasia :* (coagulo-deficiency disease) purpura, agranulocytosis etc.
   a. Raised arterial pressure : Hypertension commonest cause due to arterio sclerosis, chronic nephritis etc.
   b. Raised Venous pressure.
      i) Mitral stenosis
      ii) Whooping cough
      iii) Mediastinal tumours; vena caval syndrome
      iv) Pericardial effusion
6. *Endocrinal :* Vicarious menstruation
7. *Deficiency disease :* Malnutrition. Vit K & Vit C deficiency
8. *Environmental :* Pressure changes in high altitude.
9. *Toxic :* Uraemia, toxaemia etc.

**Epistaxis in different age groups :**

Epistaxis can occur in any age group, but aetiology varies :

1. *Children :* Common causes are injury nose, nose-picking, exanthematous fevers, foreign body nose, diphtheretic rhinitis, enlarged adenoids etc.
2. *Adolescents and young adult :* Juvenile nasopharyngeal angiofibroma (in male), trauma etc.
3. *Adult :* Acute and chronic sinusitis, injury nose (playing, boxing etc), head injury, specific rhinitis etc.
4. *Elderly :* Hypertension; malignant growth of the nose, paranasal sinuses and nasopharynx etc.

***Common sites of epistaxis :***

1. Little's area is the *commonest* (80%), particularly in children.
2. Above the middle turbinate from anterior ethmoid artery.
3. Middle meatus and post. part of lateral wall—from sphenopalatine artery.

## TREATMENT OF CHOICE

***Nasal & Facial Trauma***

* Nasal bones manipulation—*Walsham's forceps to be used.*
* Nasal septum manipulation—*Asche's forceps to be used.*
* Deviated nasal septum—*Submucous resection.*
* Frontal sinus fracture—*Adequate reduction of broken fragments to reduce the CSF leakage* (SOS—exploration & reduction to prevent deformity).
* Blow-out fracture—*Exploration of orbit & reconstruction of orbital floor with sialastic.*
* Zygomatic fracture—*Operative reduction* (closed or open technique).
* Septal perforation—*Split-skin graft or septal mucoperichondrial flaps or buccal flaps used to close the perforation site.*

***Epistaxis***

* First aid measures—*Sitting patient forwards & pinching nostril tight : Ice is sucked & put over forehead. Insertion of pledget of cotton wool soaked in adrenaline solution to nostril.*
* Patient presents with a non-acute recurrent epistaxis & blood vessel can be seen — *Cauterization of blood vessel by silver nitrate, trichloracetic acid, chromic acid, bead or electric cautery.* (SOS—Supportive measures of resuscitation).
* If blood vessels either cannot be seen or cauterized—BIPP (*Bismuth Iodoform Pataffin Paste).* Soaked ribbon gauze nasal pack for 48 hours (either anterior or posterior).
* Haemorrhage in epistaxis if not controlled by packing & cautery—Arterial ligature.

* Epistaxis in hereditary haemorrhagic telangiectasia woman—Oestrogen therapy.
* Hereditary haemorrhagic telangiectasia with epistaxis—Septodermaplasty (Radiation—as last resort).

**Acute Sinusitis**

* Uncomplicated common cold & influenza—Supportive measures (salicylates to control pyrexia).
* If acute sinusitis does not resolve with simple measures—Intranasal antrostomy. (Drainage of frontal sinus—trephine i.e. external drainage through a roof or orbit incision; ethmoid sinus —drain spontaneously; Sphenoiditis—*Anterior sphenoidotomy).*
* Orbital cellulitis—Broad spectrum systemic antibiotic + intranasal decongestants + Surgical drainage through superomedial incision of orbit.
* Frontal osteomyelitis (Pott's puffy tumour)—Surgical drainage through floor of the frontal sinus.
* Meningitis & cavernous sinus thrombosis—High levels of broad-spectrum antibiotics (systemically).

**Chronic Rhinitis**

* Chronic rhinitis—least invasive treatment —*Cautery.*
* Chronic rhinitis with enormous sized turbinates—*Turbinoplasty.*
* Rhinitis medicamentosa—Immediate cessation of decongestant & replacement by Nasal or systemic steroids (SOS—turbinectomy).
* Vestibulitis—Avoidance of touching vestibule with dirty finger nails + use of topical antibiotics.
* Atrophic rhinitis—Airway narrowing operation (Teflon injection into inferior turbinate or medializing the lateral wall of nostril + Recurrent steam inhalations + instillation of petroleum jelly + 25% glucose in glycerol drops).
* Rhinitis sicca—Petroleum jelly + repeated steam inhalations + 25% glucose in glycerol drops.

**Chronic Sinusitis**

* Chronic maxillary sinusitis—*Surgical treatment* (antral lavage, intranasal antrostomy).

* Chronic long standing cases or where antral lavage & intranasal antrostomy failed to cure chronic maxillary sinusitis—*Caldwell-Luc operation.*
* Chronic frontal sinusitis—Osteoplastic frontal flap operation.
* Chronic ethmoidal sinusitis—Endoscopic surgery of ethmoids or external, intranasal & transantral approach (via Caldwell-Luc incision).
* Chronic sphenoid sinusitis—Surgery carried out through external ethmoidectomy approach, or intranasal approach.
* Symptomatic cysts of maxillary sinus (Embryological cysts; follicular & Radicular dental cysts) — *Exanteration.*
* Oroantral fistula—Immediate suture at the time of dental treatment (in the absence of retained roof).
* Oroantral fistula with sinus infection—Radical antrostomy under antibiotic cover, and fistula repair by mucoperiosteal flap.

**Allergic rhinitis & nasal polyps**

* Allergic rhinitis—
    * Medical treatment—Decongestants, oral antihistamines, hyposensitization, sodium chromoglycate & steroids.
    * Surgical treatment—Turbinate surgery of Vidian neurectomy.
    * Nasal polyps—*Polypectomy* + Steroid spray indefinitely (to prevent recurrences).
    * Recurrent nasal polyps—Repeated polypectomy (SOS—ethmoidectomy).
    * Choanal polyp—Complete removal of polyp + Removal of the lining of the sinus (to avoid recurrence).

**Catarrhal child**

* Nasal catarrh associated with mucopurulent discharge and attacks of otitis media in children.
* Nasal catarrh associated with recurrent attacks of acute tonsillitis—Tonsillectomy.
* Congenital bilateral choanal atresia in infants—Perforation of occlusion by opened widely for membrane & openly by a proof puncture trocar & canula for osseous.

**Nasal granuloma :**

* Syphilis—Penicillin (treatment of choice) + Nose cleansed by frequent douching & removal of loose sequestra.
* Lupus vulgaris & Tuberculosis—Antituberculous chemotherapy.
* Wegener's granuloma—Corticosteroids + Immunosuppressive agents (Cyclophosphamide & Azathioprin).
* Stewart's granuloma—Radiotherapy.

**Fungal infections of Nose :**

* Rhinosporidiosis—Wide excision.

**Cancer of nose & sinuses**

* Transitional-cell carcinoma—Excision through lateral rhinotomy followed by Radiotherapy.
* Tumours of septum—Radiotherapy.
* Recurrent tumours of septum —Total rhinectomy & removal of the central segment of upper lip with reconstruction by forehead flap & Abbe lip flap.

---

## NOSE & SINUSES OPERATIONS

---

1. ***Submucous resection of the septum (SMR)***—Involves incising the mucoperichondrium parallel but 1.25 cm behind the columella & elevating the mucoperichondrium flap of the septal cartilage.

*Indications :*

* Total or subtotal obstruction of one nasal cavity by a bony or cartilaginous deflection.
* Obstruction to the drainage of PNS.
* External deformity
* Mouth breathing
* As on operation of access to a bleeding point in cases of epistaxis.
* As an operation of access to the patient's ethmoid or sphenoid sinuses.

*Contraindications :*

* Before the age of 18
* Elderly persons
* Presence of acute infection
* Specific infection like syphilis & tuberculosis

*Complications:*

* Haemorrhage
* Septal haematoma
* Septal perforation
* Septal abscess
* Flappy septum
* Neuralgic pain
* Adhesion of septum with lateral wall of nose.
* Collapse of dorsum of nose.
* Intracranial complications—

  Meningitis

  Cavernous sinus thrombosis

2. ***Trans-sphenoidal Hypophysectomy :***

   Removal of pituitary gland through transphenoidal route.

*Indications :*

* Normal pituitary gland removal—

  Disseminated or endocrine-dependent breast cancer.

  Gross proliferative new vessel formation in diabetic retinopathy (not amenable to laser therapy).
* *Pituitary adenomas associated with*—Acromegaly, Cushing's disease, panhypopituitarism, Nelson's syndrome, hyperprolactinemic hypoglonadism in woman.

***Contraindications :***

* Nose & sinus infection
* Superior vena cava block
* Hepatic failure
* Poor pneumatization of sphenoidal sinus

3. ***Antral Puncture (Proof-puncture) and wash-out :*** Maxillary antrum is punctured and washed out through the inferior means for diagnostic and therapeutic purpose.

*Indications :*

* Chronic suppurative maxillary sinusitis for diagnostic and therapeutic purpose.
* In some cases of acute maxillary sinusitis, where medical treatment has failed.

* Indwelling of polythene tube in the maxillary sinus in chronic sinusitis for subsequent wash-out.
* Cytology from maxillary sinus.
* Oro-antral fistula with sinusitis.

*Complications :*

* Puncture of the orbital floor would result in orbital injury or cellulitis.
* Puncture of posterior wall may result in swelling of the cheek through pterygo-maxillary fissure.
* Puncture into the cheek by too anterior placement, would result in cellulitis of the face.
* Air-embolism
* Haemorrhage (epistaxis) due to injury of a vessel.

**4. *Intranasal Antrostomy :***

*Definition :* It is the operation in which a permanent enlarged opening is made in the inferior meatus for drainage of the maxillary sinus (anterior to the site of antral puncture).

*Anaesthesia :* Local anaesthesia is usual but in some apprehensive cases general anaesthesia has to be administered.

*Indications :*

1. Chronic suppurative maxillary sinusitis, when repeated antral puncture has failed to clear-up pus.
2. In some cases, biopsy can be taken through the opening.
3. After reduction of fracture of the maxilla.
4. Following Caldwell Luc operation.
5. Oro-antral fistula.
6. Trans-antral ethmoidectomy.
7. Also performed before sinoscopy.

**5. *Caldwell-luc Operation (Radical antrostomy) :***

Maxillary antrum is opened through canine fossa by sublabial approach and diseases pathology is thoroughly removed from antral cavity.

*Indications :*

1. Chronic maxillary sinusitis, where repeated antral-wash has failed.
2. Recurrent anto-choanal polyp.
3. Biopsy from maxillary antrum.
4. Foreign body in maxillary antrum.
5. Reduction of fracture of the maxilla.
6. Trans-antral ethmoidectomy.
7. Ligation of the maxillary artery.
8. Oro-antral fistula.
9. Mucocele of the maxillary sinus.
10. Osteoma or other benign tumours of the maxillary sinus.

*Complications :*

1. Injury to the infra-orbital nerve.
2. Injury to the root of the teeth.
3. Haemorrhage.
4. Facial cellulitis.
5. Venous sinus thrombosis (Cavernous sinus).

**6. *External frontal operation :***

The frontal sinus is approached directly through floor by Howarth's incision keeping the anterior wall intact.

*Indications :*

1. Chronic suppurative frontal sinusitis.
2. Mucocele of the frontal sinus
3. Pyocele of the frontal sinus
4. Foreign body in the frontal sinus.
5. Osteoma of the frontal sinus.

*Complications :*

1. Orbital cellulitis.
2. Meningitis
3. Cavernous sinus thrombosis.
4. Epistaxis.

**7.** ***External ethmoidectomy operation :***

The approach is through a curved incision from medial third under the eye-brow to below the inner canthus of the eye on the side of the nose. The diseased ethmoidal cells and polyps are remove thoroughly.

**8.** ***Septoplasty :***

This is the modern method of surgical treatment of deviated nasal septum. The operation is approached through concave side.

*Indications :*

1. In children and adolescents requiring septal surgery.
2. Anterior cartilaginous deformity
3. Anterior septal dislocation
4. Along with rhinoplasty

This is a conservative form of surgery with minimum excision of cartilage and bone. The displaced cartilage is carefully separated by tunneling and replaced back to position by varieties of techniques.

# PHARYNX

## MEMBRANOUS LESIONS IN THE PHARYNX

The diseaes producing membranous lesions in the pharynx are :

1. Acute follicular tonsillitis
2. Acute diphtheric pharyngitis
3. Vincent's angina
4. Fungus infection
5. Infectious mononucleosis
6. Agranulocytic angina (Agranulocytosis)
7. Acute streptococcal pharyngitis
8. Keratosis pharyngis

## INVESTIGATIONS OF CHOICE

| | |
|---|---|
| * Acute tonsilitis | Throat swab for isolation & c/s of organisms |
| * Tuberculosis of tonsil | Histopathology of tonsil |
| * Infectious mononucliosis (Glandular fever) | Blood film—atypical large mononuclear cells; TWBC—10.0-20.0 x $10^9/1$; positive Monospot test. |
| * Moniliasis (Thrush) | Salivary washings for causative fungi. |
| * Syphilis of the pharynx | Serological tests & biopsy of pharynx. |
| * Scleroma of the pharynx | Hard infiltrations on section—Hyaline bodies & Mikulicz cells & from lesions—diplobacillus. |
| * Leprosy of the pharynx | Bacilli from nasal discharge & biopsy of nodule. |
| * Sarcoidosis of the pharynx | Biopsy & positive Kveim-test. |

| | | |
|---|---|---|
| * | Nasopharyngeal carcinoma | Radiography—(Tomogram—for bone destruction. CT scan—for tumour extension, MRI—for soft-tissue involvement, and Biopsy). |
| * | Oropharyngeal tumours | Biopsy & CT scan for parapharyngeal tumour extension. |
| * | Hypopharyngeal tumours | Barium swallow (the key investigation). |

## TREATMENT OF CHOICE

**Infections of the pharynx**

* Adenoid hypertrophy—not well marked & symptoms are slight—Simple breathing exercises & reassurance (No surgical treatment).
* Adenoid hypertrophy with the presence of one or more cardinal symptoms—Adenoidectomy.
* Acute tonsillitis—Bed rest + Aspirin + Antibiotics + Administration of fluids.
* Peritonsillar abscess (Quinsy)—Systemic penicillin.
* If antibiotics fails to relieve Quinsy in 24-48 hours—Incision & Drainage + Continuation of penicillin (until complete resolution).
* Chronic tonsillitis (recurrent)—Tonsillectomy.
* Acute infection of the lingual tonsil—Antibiotics.
* Chronic enlargement of the lingual tonsil—Cryo-surgery
* Calculus of the tonsils—Removal with a probe
* Calculus of the tonsil with recurrent infections—Tonsillectomy.
* Retention cyst of the tonsil—Reassurance.
* Acute pharyngitis—No treatment (SOS—Aspirin; in presence of pyrexia—Antibiotics).
* Chronic pharyngitis —Avoidance of tobacco, wearing a mask etc.

**Neck space infections**

* Retropharyngeal abscess in infants—Incision & Drainage.
* Retropharyngeal abscess in adults—Incision & Drainage (incision over posterior borders of sternomastoid) + Antituberculous therapy.

* Parapharyngeal abscess—Incision & Drainage (vertical incision over anterior border of sternomastoid) + Antibiotics.
* Ludwig's angina (submandibular space infection)—Antibiotics.

**Tumours of the nasopharynx**

* Nasopharyngeal carcinoma & Lymphoma—Radiotherapy (treatment of choice) and neck should be included in the field.
* Nasopharyngeal carcinoma where lymph nodes are not controlled by radiation or where enlarged nodes appear after the primary has been controlled—Radical neck dissection surgery.
* Recurrence of the primary tumour of nasopharyngeal carcinoma—Further course of radiation.
* Angiofibroma of the nasopharynx with bone destruction & with a liberal cross- circulation at the skull base—Embolizaton followed by radiotherapy (other cases—Surgery is the treatment of choice).

**Tumours of the oropharynx :**

* Tonsil carcinoma :
  * Without palpable neck nodes—Irradiation (primary treatment)
  * With palpable neck nodes—Commando operation (Removal of fauces, part of palate & base of tongue, part of mandible and radical neck dissection) + Reconstruction of pharynx with pectoralis major myocutaneous flap.

**Tumours of the hypopharynx :**

* Small pyriform fossa carcinoma & does not involve the postcricoid region and without palpable nodes—Radiotherapy (primary treatment).
* Small pyriform fossa carcinoma and does not invole the postcricoid region but nodes palpable or recurrent carcinoma—total laryngopharyngectomy+Reconstruction either with free segment of jejunum & small-vessel anastomosis or pectoralis major myocutaneous flap.

# PHARYNX OPERATIONS

I. ***Tonsillectomy***

*Indications :*

* Repeated acute tonsillitis (> 3 attacks a year).
* Repeated sore throats (> 4 to 6 times a year or more) association with sore throats or acute tonsillitis.
* One attack of peritonsillar abscess (quinsy).
* Recurrent middle-ear infection in association with sore throats or acute tonsillitis.
* Chronic tonsillitis (when other treatment gives no relief).
* Chronic infection with β-haemolytic streptococci or diphtheria organisms in carriers.
* Secondary effects in other organs.
* Tuberculous cervical adenitis is adversely affected by suppurative chronic infection.
* Chronic infection with gross hypertrophy causing gross obstruction to breathing, swallowing & speaking.
* As a preliminary stage to operation for cleft palate.
* In avulsion of glossopharyngeal nerve & removal of styloid process for neuralgia (through pharyngeal route).
* As a precautionary & diagnostic measure for suspicion of malignancy of tonsil

*Contraindications :*

* There are no absolute contraindications for tonsillectomy.
* Allergic rhinitis & Asthma.
* Bleeding tendency
* Epidemics of any infectious disease (especially poliomyelitis).

*Choice of operation :*

* Guillotine method—it is shorter, but no longer used.
* Dissection method—it is the method of choice.

*Complications :*

* Reactionary haemorrhage (occurs within a few hours of the operation).
* Infection
* Pain on swallowing (for the 1st week).
* Speech is affected (until slough separates).
* Otitis media
* Oedema of soft palate.
* Cervical lymphadenitis
* Parapharyngeal abscess
* Septicaemia
* Pneumonia or lung abscess
* Flare-up of distant infections
* Dental injuries

**II.** ***Adenoidectomy :***

*Indications :*

* If the size of adenoids is interfering with —nasal or auditory tube ventilation, speech or feeding.
* Chronic infection is the cause of repeated upper respiratory tract infection—recurrent otitis media, chronic catarrh, headache, nocturnal cough or lethargy.
* Normal obstruction associated with infection.
* Along with myringotomy & grommet insertion in secretory otitis media.
* Along with antral lavage in maxillary sinusitis.
* Along with tonsillectomy as a specific indication.

*Contraindications :*

* Blood dyscrasia
* Jaundice
* Acute infection

*Complications :*

* Primary haemorrhage (during operation)

* Reactionary haemorrhage
* Secondary haemorrhage (occurs 5-10 post- operative days).
* Unusual haemorrhage (due to aberrant vessels injury)
* Incomplete removal—Recurrence
* Hypernasality (rhinolalia aperta).
* Acute otitis media
* Chronic nasopharyngitis.
* Granular pharyngitis.

# EPONYMS IN E.N.T.

***Adenoid facies :*** Crowded teeth, high-arched palate, underdeveloped nostrils

***Adler bodies :*** Deposits of mucopolysaccharide found in neutrophils of the patients with Hurler's syndrome.

***Antoni's type A and type B :***

Type-I : Downward protrusion of the long, thin, cerebellar tonsils through the foramen magnus

Type-II : Protrusion of the inferior cerebellar vermis through the foramen.

Type-III : Bony occipital defect with descent of the entire cerebellum.

Type-IV : Cerebellar hypoplasia.

***Abrikossoffs tumor*** (granular cell myoblastoma) : Causes pseudoepithelial hyperplasia in the larynx, the site most favoured in the larynx being the posterior half of the vocal cord. Three percent of granular cell myoblastoma progress to malignancy. In order of decreasing frequency of involvement, the granular cell myoblastoma occurs in tongue, skin breast subcutaneous tissue, and respiratory tract.

***Arnold's ganglion :*** Otic ganglion.

***Achoff body :*** Rheumatic nodule found in rheumatic disease.

***Ballet's sign*** : Paralysis of voluntary movements of the eyeball with preservation of the automatic movements. Sometimes this sign is present with exophthalmic goiter and hysteria.

***Bechterew's symptom :*** Paralysis of facial muscles limited to automatic movements. The power of voluntary movement is retained.

***Bednar's aphthae :*** Symmetrical excoriations of the hard palate in the region of the pterygoid plates due to sucking the thumb, foreign objects, or scalding.

***Bezold's abscess :*** Abscess in the sternocleidomastoid muscle secondary to perforation of the tip of the mastoid by infection.

***Blandin, gland of :*** A minor salivary gland situated in the anterior portion of the tongue.

***Brooke's tumor :***(epithelioma adenoid cystica) : It originates from the hair follicles in the external auditory canal and auricle. It is of basal cell origin. Treatment is local resection.

***Broyle's ligament :*** Anterior commissure ligament of the larynx.

***Brudzinski's sign :*** With meningitis passive flexion of the leg on one side causes a similar movement to occur in the opposite leg. Passive flexion of the neck brings about flexion of the legs as well.

***"Brunner's abscess :*** Abscess of the posterior floor of the mouth.

***Bruns sign :*** A gurgling is heard in a neck mass. It suggests a laryngocele.

***Carhart's notch :*** Maximum dip at 2000 kHz (bone conduction) seen in patient with otosclerosis.

***Charcot-Leyden crystals :*** Crystals in the shape of elongated double pyramids, composed of spermine phosphates and present in the sputum of asthmatic patients. Synonyms are Charcot Newman crystals, Charcot-Robin crystals.

***Charcot's triad :*** The nystagmus, scanning speech, and intention tremor seen in multiple sclerosis.

***Cherubism :*** Familial, with the age of predilection between 2 and 5 years. It is characterized by giant cell reparative granuloma causing cystic lesions in the posterior rami of the mandible. The lesions are usually symetrical. It is a self-limiting disease with remissions after puberty. The maxilla also may be involved.

***Chvostek's sign :*** It is the facial twitch obtained by tapping the distribution of the facial nerve. It is indicative of hypocalcemia and is the most reliable test for hypocalcemia.

***Curschmann's spirals :*** Spirally twisted masses of mucus present in the sputum of bronchial asthmatic patients.

***Demarquay's sign :*** Absence of elevation of the larynx during deglutition. It is said to indicate syphilitic induration of the trachea.

***Di Sant' Agnese test :*** It measures the elevated sodium and chloride in the sweat of cystic fibrotic children.

***Dupre's sign*** : Meningism.

***Ebner, gustatory glands of*** : These glands are the minor salivary glands near the circumvallate papillae.

***Escherich's sign :*** In hypoparathyroidism, tapping of the skin at the angle of the mouth causes protrusion of the lips.

***Galen's anastomosis :*** An anastomosis between the superior laryngeal nerve and the recurrent laryngeal nerve.

***Goodwin's tumor :*** Benign lymphoepithelioma.

***Griesinger's sign :*** Edema of the tip of the mastoid in thrombosis of the sigmoid sinus.

***Guttman's test*** : In the normal subject, frontal pressure on the thyroid cartilage lowers the tone of voice produced, whereas lateral pressure produces a higher tone of voice. The opposite is true with paralysis of the cricothyroid muscle.

***Guyton's sign*** : The XII nerve lies directly upon the external carotid artery, whereby this vessel may be distinguished from the internal carotid artery. (The safer way prior to ligation of the external carotid artery is to identify the first few branches of the external carotid artery).

*Henle, glands of* : They are the small glands situated in the areolar tissue between the buccopharyngeal fascia anteriorly and the prevertebral fascia posteriorly. Infection of these glands can lead to retropharyngeal abscess. Because these glands atrophy at the age of 5, retropharyngeal abscess is less likely to occur after that age.

***Hennebert's sign :*** The presence of a positive fistula test in the absence of an obvious fistula is called Hennerbert's sign. The patient has a normal-appearing tympanic membrane and external auditory canal. The nystagmus is more marked upon application of negative pressure. This sign is present with congenital syphilis and is believed to be due to an excessively mobile footplate or caused by motion of the saccule mediated by fibrosis between the footplate and the saccule.

***Hering-Breuter reflex :*** It is respiratory reflex from pulmonary stretch receptors. Inflation of the lungs sends an inhibitory impulse to the central nervous system via the vagus nerve to stop inspiration. Similarly, deflation of the lungs sends an impulse to stop expiration. The action is the Hering-Breuer reflex.

***Kernig's sign :*** When the subject lies on his back with the thigh at a right angle to the trunk, straightening of the leg (extending the leg) elicits pain, supposedly owing to the pull on the inflammed lumbosacral nerve roots. This sign is present with meningitis.

***Kiesselbach's plexus :*** This area is in the anterior septum where the capillaries merge. It is often the site of anterior epistaxis. It also been referred to as *Little's area.*

***Koplil's spots :*** Pale round spots on oral mucosa, conjunctiva and lacrimal caruncle, seen in the early stages of measles.

***Krause's nodes :*** They are the nodes in the jugular foramen.

***Lhermitte's sign :*** Patient develop sensory deficits and complain of "electric shocks" radiating down the back and into the extremities after neck flexion. It occurs 2 to 4 months after completion of radiation therapy to the CNS or spinal canal and is classified as an early transient thrombophlebitis.

***Little-Crowe test :*** Used in the diagnosis of unilateral lateral sinus thrombophlebitis. Digital compression of the opposite internal jugular vein causes the retinal veins to dilate.

***Little's area :*** See Kiesselpach's plexuses.

***Ludwig's angina :*** Ac. inflammatory, process beginning on floor of mouth that invades mylohyoid and submandibular space.

***Luschka pouch :*** See Thronwalt's cyst

***Macus Gunn's phenomenon :*** Unilateral ptosis of the eyelid with exaggerated opening of the eye during movements of the mandible.

***Marjolin's ulcer :*** It is carcinoma that arises at the site of an old burn scar. It is a well differentiated squamous cell carcinoma that is aggressive and metastasizes rapidly.

***Meckel's ganglion :*** Sphenopalatine ganglion.

***Mikulicz's cells :*** These cells are macrophages in rhinoscleroma. (*Russel bodies,* which are eosinophilic, round structures associated with plasma cells, also are found with rhinoscleroma).

***Mollaret-Debre test :*** This test is performed for cat-scratch fever.

***Morgagni, sinus of :*** A dehiscence of the superior constrictor muscle and the buccopharyngeal fascia where the eustachian tube opens.

***Morgagni, ventricle of :*** It separates the quadrangular membrane from the conus elasticus in the larynx.

***Nikolsky's sign :*** Detachment of the sheets of the superficial epithelial layers when any traction is applied over the surface of the epithelial involvement in pemphigus is characteristic of Nikolsky's sign. Pemphigus involves the intraepithelial layer, whereas pemphigoid involves the subepithelial layer. The former is a lethal disease in many instances.

***Oliver-Cardarelli sign :*** Reversion of the larynx and trachea is synchronous with cardiac systole in cases of aneurysm of the arch of the aorta or in cases of a tumor in the region.

***Parinaud's sign :*** Extraocular muscle impairment with decreased upward gaze and ptosis seen in association with pinealomas and other lesions of the tectum.

***Paul-Bunnel test :*** It measures the elevated heterophile titer of infectious mononucleosis.

***Rathke's pouch :*** See Thornwaldt's cyst.

***Reinke's tumor :*** It is a "soft" tumor variant of lymphoepithelioma in which the lymphocytes predominate. (With the hard tumor the epithelial cells predominate; it is called *Schmincke's tumor).*

***Rhomberg's sign :*** If a patient standing with feet together "falls" when he closes his eyes, the Rhomberg test is positive. It is indicative of either abnormal proprioception or abnormal vestibular function. It does not necessarily distinguish central from peripheral lesions. Cerebellar function is not tested by this test.

***Rosenbach's sign :*** Fine tremor of the closed eyelids seen in hyperthyroidism and hysteria.

***Rouvier's sign :*** Lateral retropharyngeal node. It is common target of metastasis in nasopharyngeal carcinoma.

***Russell's bodies :*** Eosinophilic, round structures, associated with plasma cells found in rhinoscleroma.

***Santorini's fissures :*** Fissures in the anterior bony external auditory canal leading to the parotid region.

***Santorini's tumor :*** The "hard" variant of lymphoepithelioma in which the epithelial cells predominate.

***Schneiderian mucosa :*** Pseudostratified ciliated columnar mucosa of the nose.

***Seligmuller's sign :***Contraction of the pupil on the affected side in facial neuralgia.

***Semon' sign :*** A law stating that injury in the recurrent laryngeal nerve results in paralysis of the abductor muscle of the larynx (cricoarytenoid posticus) before paralysis of the abductor muscles. During recovery the abductor recovers before the abductor.

***Straus' sign :*** With facial paralysis the lesion is peripheral if injection of pilocarpine is followed by sweating on the affected side later than on the normal side.

***Sulkowitch's test :*** It determines an increase in calciuria.

***Tobey-Ayer-Queckenstedt test :*** Used in the diagnosis of unilateral and bilateral sinus thrombophlebitis. In cases where the lateral sinus is obstructed on one side, compression of the jugular vein on the intact side causes a rise in CSF pressure, whereas compression of the obstructed side does not raise the CSF pressure.

***Thornwaldt's cyst :*** A depression exists in the nasopharyngeal vault that is a remnants of the pouch of Luschka. When this depression becomes infected, Thronwaldt's cyst results. In the early embryo, this area has connection between the notochord and endoderm. Thornwaldt's cyst is lined with respiratory epithelium with some squamous metaplasia. Anterior to this pit, the path taken by Rathke's pouch sometimes persists as the craniopharyngeal canal, running from the sella turcica through the body of the sphenoid to an opening on the undersurface of the skull.

***Toynbee's law :*** When CNS complications arise in chronic otitis media, the lateral sinus and cerebellum are involved in mastoiditis, whereas the cerebrum alone is involved in instances of cholesteatoma of the attic.

***Trousseau's sign :*** With hypocalcemia tourniquet placed around the arm causes tetany.

***Tullo's phenomenon :*** This phenomenon is said to be present when a loud noise precipitates vertigo. It can be present in congenital syphilis, with a semicircular canal fistula, or in postfenestration patient if the footplate is mobile. The tympanic membrane and ossicular chain must be intact with a mobile footplate.

***Wartenberg's sign :***Intense pruritus of the tip of the nose and nostril indicates cerebral tumor.

***Warthin-Finkelday giant cells :*** They are found in the lymphoid with measles.

***Weber's glands :*** These glands are minor salivary glands in the superior pole of the tonsil.

***Xeroderma pigmentosa :*** Hereditary precancerous condition that begins during early childhood. These patients die at puberty.

***Zaufal's sign :*** Saddle nose.

# NAMED SYNDROMES

| *Name* | *Symptoms & Signs* | *Treatment* |
|---|---|---|
| **Albright's Syndrome** | It is an asymmetric disease of bones of face (osteitis fibrosa cystica) with melanotic pigmentation of skin and sexual precocity. | Facial asymmetry can be corrected by surgical procedure. |
| **Abrich's Syndrome** | Chronic eczema , CSOM. Anaemia, Thrombocytic purpura. | |
| **Alport's Syndrome** | Presenile familial nerve deafness (Bilateral). Congenital haemorrhagic nephritis. Keratoconus and cataracts. | Pure tone audiometry and urine examination. Hearing aid |
| **Arnold-Chiari Syndrome of Malformation** | Stridor, cough due to aspiration, difficulty in feeding Bilateral vocal cord analysis, Hydrocephalus, Meningomyelocele. | Treatment of the cause Tracheostomy in emergency cases |
| **Ascher's Syndrome** | Blepharochalasis, (acquired atrophy of skin of the upper eye-lid). Adenoma of thyroid gland. Redundancy of the mucous membrane and submucous tissue of upper lip. | |
| **Avilles' Syndrome** | Results due to lesion in nucleus ambigus or vagus nerve or cranial accessory contralateral loss of pain and due to spinothalamic destruction. Dysphagia due to laryngeal and pharyngeal paralysis, nasal regurgitation and Rhinolalia. | Treatment of the cause |

(Contd.......)

## NAMED SYNDROMES (Contd....)

| *Name* | *Symptoms & Signs* | *Treatment* |
|---|---|---|
| | due to paralysis of soft palate. The symptoms may be progressive in that the palatal paralysis may not develop before the laryngeal paralysis. The cause is usually avascular or inflammatory lesions in the medulla, but the diseases involving the vagus nerve above the level of nodose ganglion will cause similar paralysis.<br>Hoarseness of voice.<br>Nasal Twang with regurgitation.<br>Palato-Laryngeal hemiplegia. | |
| **Barany's Syndrome** | Giddiness, Deafness, Tinnitus and pain in the back of the head.<br>Vertigo and nystagmus most marked on looking to healthy side.<br>Falling and past pointing to diseased side. | Labyrinthine sedatives, antibiotics |
| **Behcet's Syndrome** | Massive and indulent ulceration of mucous membranes and sometimes skin of anogenital region.<br>Inflammation of eyes, Pain & Loss of weight.<br>Ulcerations of mucous membrane and skin<br>Iritis, hypopyon, choroiditis, retinitis. | Steroids |

(Contd.......)

## NAMED SYNDROMES (Contd....)

| *Name* | *Symptoms & Signs* | *Treatment* |
|---|---|---|
| **Brain's Syndrome** | Episodic attacks of nausea and vomiting resembling. Meniere's disease.<br>Diplopia, Vertigo, Loss of vision, Drowsiness & Disturbance of consciousness with incoherent and difficult speech.<br>Nystagmus, Ataxia, Hypotonia of limbs and Bilateral papilloedema | Treatment of cause. |
| **Cogan's Syndrome** | Pain in the eye, watering of the eye with diminution of vision, Deafness, Vertigo, Tinnitus and Nausea & vomiting.<br>Non-syphilitic interstitial keratitis with vestibulo-auditory dysfunction. | |
| **Cardio-Auditory Syndrome of Jervell and Lang-Nielsen (1957)** | Deafness, Fainting attacks.<br>Recessive deafness, ECG abnormalities, Prolonged Q-T Interval & death following syncope due to cardiac arrest or arrhythmia. | Symptomatic treatment |
| **Chorda-Tympani Syndrome** | Sweating in the submental region. | Section of the chorda-tympani nerve by endural route. |
| **Collet-Sicard Syndrome** | Hoarseness of voice, Nasal twang and regurgitation.<br>Difficult in speech & Reduced sense of taste.<br>Homolateral paralysis of tongue soft palate, larynx, neck muscles associated with diminished sensation and reduced sense of taste due to simultaneous involvement of last four cranial nerves in the region of jugular foramen. | Treatment of cause |

(Contd.......)

## NAMED SYNDROMES (Contd....)

| *Name* | *Symptoms & Signs* | *Treatment* |
|---|---|---|
| **Costen's Syndrome** | Pain in the temporomandibular joint with referred otalgia.<br>Tinnitus and feeling of muffing in the ears.<br>Mal-occlusion of Temporomandibular joint. | Correction of malocclusion |
| **Crocodile tear syndrome** | Watering of the eye while eating.<br>Gustatory lacrimation. | Resection of Tympani nerve |
| **Crouzen's Syndrome** | Deafness, Craniofacial dysostosis with small maxilla.<br>Hypoplasia of maxilla, ectropion and districhiasis.<br>Additional row of eye lashes at the inner margin.<br>Hypertelorism, Oxycephaly.<br>Bony ankylosis of stapes causing conductive deafness. | For stapes fixation stapedectomy is done. |
| **Down' Syndrome (Trisomy-21) (Mongolism)** | Mental retardation, hypotonia, craniofacial dysostosis, Congenital Heart disease, decreased acetabular and iliac angles, small penis, cryptorchidism. Simian crease, short broad hands, hypoplasia of middle phalanx of 5th finger, gap between 1st and 2nd toes. High arched palate, strabismus, broad short neck, small teeth, furrowed tongue, intestinal atresia, imperforate anus. | |
| **Duane's Syndrome** | Otic malformation, Diplopia.<br>Atresia of ear.<br>Congenital paresis of lateral rectus muscle. | Plastic surgery of ear |

(Contd.......)

## NAMED SYNDROMES (Contd....)

| *Name* | *Symptoms & Signs* | *Treatment* |
|---|---|---|
| **Dysmalia Syndrome** | Deafness, Vestibular disorder, Facial weakness and Diplopia.<br>Physical and otic malformations<br>Abducent and facial nerve paralysis. | |
| **Edward's Syndrome (Trisomy-18)** | Mental retardation, hypertonia, failure to thrive, preponderance in females, low birth weight.<br>Prominent occiput, micrognathia, low set malformed ears, congenital heart disease, mainly VSD and PDA, Horse-shoe kidney, small pelvis, cryptorchidism, inguinal hernia, Flexion deformity of fingers, equinovarus Cleft lip and palate, ocular anomalies, webbed neck. | |
| **Fran Ceschetti-Zwahlen Syndrome** | | Same as Treacher-Collin's Syndrome |
| **Frey's Syndrome (also called as Balliainger's Syndrome and Auriculotemporal Syndrome)** | Flushing and sweating of face during swallowing<br>Gustatory flushing and sweating of face about the area of auriculotemporal nerve | Resection of tympanic nerve |
| **Gardener's Syndrome** | Multiple colonic polyposis which are premalignant<br>Generalised multiple soft tissue swellings in the form of fibromas, lipomas, neurofibromas<br>Multiple osteomas of facial bones | |

(Contd.......)

## NAMED SYNDROMES (Contd....)

| *Name* | *Symptoms & Signs* | *Treatment* |
|---|---|---|
| **Goldenhar's Syndrome** | Otic anomalies like Atresia of ear.<br>Facial anomalies like Congenital eyelid dermoids, Notching of upper eyelid<br>Vertebral anomalies (cervical) | Plastic surgery of ear and face. |
| **Gradenigo's Syndrome** | Otorrhoa, Diplopia, Retro-orbital pain or Facial pain.<br>Abducent nerve palsy<br>Pain along trigeminal nerve, more retro-orbital. | Radical mastoidectomy with drainage of abscess from petrous apex. |
| **Grische's Syndrome** | Neck stiffness, Palpitations.<br>Stiffness of neck, opisthotonos, tachycardia, painful contracture of cervical muscles. | No pillows to be used, Muscle relaxants and sedatives. |
| **Heerfordt's Syndrome** | Swelling of parotid gland, Fever, Pain and weakness.<br>Enlarged parotid gland, Iridocyclitis and Pyrexia with paralysis of one or more cranial nerves usually facial paralysis. Boeck's sarcoidosis involving mucous membrane of upper respiratory tract. | Treatment of the cause and steroids |
| **Horner's Syndrome** | Miosis, Apparent enophthalmos, Narrowing of palpebral fissure due to ptosis. Hyperaemia of cheek & Absence of facial sweating on one side of face due to absence of sympathetic innervation (anhydrosis). | |

(Contd......)

## NAMED SYNDROMES (Contd....)

| *Name* | *Symptoms & Signs* | *Treatment* |
|---|---|---|
| **Hughlings Jackson's Syndrome** | Hoarseness of voice<br>Difficulty in speech<br>Nasal twang and nasal regurgitation.<br>Homolateral paralysis of tongue, soft palate, larynx and neck muscles. | Treatment of cause. |
| **Hurler's Syndrome** | Deafness, Visual disturbance and Cutaneous lesions.<br>Hereditary conductive deafness<br>Skeletal deformities<br>Hepatosplenomegaly<br>CNS and CVS changes (Aortic incompetance)<br>Inguinal and umbilical hernias<br>Cutaneous abnormalities<br>Corneal opacities. | |
| **Jackod's Syndrome** | Visual disturbance, Retro-orbital pain<br>Blindness, Ophthalmoplegia and<br>Pain in the distribution of 5th cranial nerve. | Radiotherapy |
| **Kartagener's Syndrome** | Nasal discharge, mild headache<br>Sinusitis, Dextrocardia, Cong. Bronchiectasis,<br>Sinus inversus and Cystic fibrosis of Pancreas. | |
| **Klinkert's Syndrome** | It is paralysis of recurrent laryngeal nerve and phrenic nerve.<br>Sympathetic paralysis may also be associated. | |

(Contd.....)

## NAMED SYNDROMES (Contd....)

| *Name* | *Symptoms & Signs* | *Treatment* |
|---|---|---|
| **Klippel-Feil Syndrome** | Deafness, Atresia of ear<br>Congenital hereditary deafness<br>Congenital short neck due to fusion of cervical and thoracic vertebrae. Low hair line extending to back. | |
| **Laurence-Moon Biedl Syndrome** | Visual disturbances, Gait disturbances<br>Voice disorders (remains highpitch).<br>Always familial but never hereditary.<br>Pigmentary degeneration of Retina.<br>Mental retardation<br>Hypogenitalism, Polydactyly, Obesity & Cerebellar ataxia and pituitary dysfunction. | Male harmones. |
| **Lermoyez Syndrome** | Deafness and tinnitus precedes an attack of vertigo after which there is immediate improvement in hearing.<br>Perceptive deafness, Nystagmus | Antihistamines e.g. Phenargan<br>Vasodilators e.g. Nicotinic acid. |
| **Marfan's Syndrome** | Deafness, Diplopia<br>High arched palate, Perceptive deafness, Convergent squint, Long tappering fingers & some toes are bigger, some are small. | |

(Contd.......)

## NAMED SYNDROMES (Contd....)

| *Name* | *Symptoms & Signs* | *Treatment* |
|---|---|---|
| **Melkersson's Syndrome** | Bilateral facial weakness (may be familial), Swelling of the upper lip.<br>Peripheral facial nerve palsy often bilateral<br>Angioneurotic oedema of face especially upper lip<br>Lingua-Plicatea (Rosenthal's symptoms) i.e. congenital fissured or furrowed tongue. | Same as Bell's Palsy (steroids and electric stimulation of facial nerve on paralysed side). |
| **Meniere's Syndrome** | Paroxysmal attacks of vertigo, Deafness and Tinnitus, Heaviness in head and Nausea and vomiting.<br>Nystagmus present during the attacks of vertigo<br>Perceptive deafness | Vasodilators like Nicothinic acid 100 mg. tds, Diuretics, Tranquilizers Labyrinthine sedatives e.g. Stemetil-5 tds. or Dramamine 50 mg tds. |
| **Mikulicz Syndrome** | Swelling of salivary glands and lacrimal glands<br>Dry mouth<br>Symmetrical enlargement of salivary glands<br>Narrowing of palpebral fissure<br>Parchment like dryness of mouth<br>Usually associated with sarcoidosis. | |
| **Moecius Syndrome** | Deafness, Perceptive in nature, Diplopia.<br>Atresia of ear, Congenital bilateral abducent palsy and aplasia of other brain-stem nuclei. | Plastic surgery of ear. |
| **Mondini Deafness** | Perceptive deafness (genetic). | Hearing aid. |
| **Morgagni's Syndrome** | Frontal intimal hyperostosis | |
| **Ortner's Syndrome** | Hoarseness of voice, Aphonia. | Treatment of mitral valve disease. |

(Contd ... )

## NAMED SYNDROMES (Contd....)

| *Name* | *Symptoms & Signs* | *Treatment* |
|---|---|---|
| **(Cardio-vocal Syndrome)** | Paralysis of left recurrent laryngeal nerve. Aphonia is present when patient turns head to left. This is due to lack of compensatory movement of right vocal cord in this position, signs of mitral valve disease. | |
| **Pancoast's Syndrome** | Neuritis pain in the arm<br>Atrophy of muscles of arm and hand<br>Associated Horner's syndrome<br>Osteolysis of ribs and vertebrae<br>Coin shadow on X-ray chest at apex of lung | |
| **Platau Syndrome (Trisomy-13)** | Mental retardation, failure to thrive, capillary haemangiomas, persistent foetal haemoglobin, Microcephaly, cleftlip and palate, midline scalp dermoids, coloboma, low-set malformed ears, deafness, congenital heart disease like PDA and VSD, polycystic kidney, bicornuate uterus, cryptorchidism, polydactyly, hyperconvex finger nails, simian crease, micrognathia, retro-flexible thumb. | |
| **Paterson-Brown-Kelly Syndrome** | Dysphagia, Glossitis with loss of papillae<br>Lips and corners of mouth are often cracked<br>Koilonychia, Splenomegaly, Anaemia and Achlorhydria | Dilatation of stricture through an oesophagoscope.<br>Blood transfusion-Iron preparations orally. |

(Contd.......)

## NAMED SYNDROMES (Contd....)

| *Name* | *Symptoms & Signs* | *Treatment* |
|---|---|---|
| **Pendred's Syndrome** | Deafness, Swelling of thyroid gland. Inherited perceptive deafness (cong. deafness, goitre in non-endemic districts). | Hearing aid. |
| **Permanent Perforation Syndrome** | Deafness and Discharge from ear. Mechanical defect in the tympanic membrane which exposes the middle ear mucosa to recurrent infections. They are confined to pars tensa and vary in size, shape and position but retain healed edge. Conductive deafness with 20-45 db loss, patient may hear better when ear is discharging due to partial closure of perforation with mucous or loading of the round window. | Keep ear dry. Myringoplasty. |
| **Peutz Syndrome (Peutz-Jegher's Syndrome** | Bleeding per rectum, Severe abdominal pain and constipation. Familial intestinal polyposis affecting mainly jejunum. Melanosis of the oral mucous membrane. | Snare the polyp by means of a fibreoptic colonoscope. |
| **Pickwickian Syndrome** | Exogenous obesity, Somnolence, Hypoventi-lation of lungs and Erythrocytosis. | |
| **Pierre Robin Syndrome** | Deaf and dumb, micrognathia Congenital deafness, mutism, Deformities of external and middle ear, Cleft lip and palate, Hypertelorism, Mandibular dysostosis, Glossoptosis. | |

(Contd.......)

## NAMED SYNDROMES (Contd....)

| *Name* | *Symptoms & Signs* | *Treatment* |
|---|---|---|
| **Ramsay Hunt Syndrome (Hunt's Syndrome)** | Pain in the ear, Loss of taste on anterior 2/3 of tongue, Facial weakness, Deafness and Vertigo.<br>Pain in the ear and palatoglossal arch Vesicles along the distribution of nerve of Wrisberg, Loss of taste on anterior 2/3 of tongue, Facial paralysis and Deafness. | |
| **Reiter's Syndrome** | Pain the eye with watering of eye<br>Pain in joint<br>Pain during micturition<br>Purulent conjunctivitis, Urethritis, Arthritis<br>ESR raised and WBC count increased. | No specific treatment<br>Eye baths and shades<br>TAB vaccine |
| **Schmidt's Syndrome** | Hoarseness of voice<br>Nasal twang with regurgitation<br>Paralysis of soft palate, pharynx, larynx, sternomastoid and trapezius muscles. | Treatment of the cause. |
| **Shy-Drager Syndrome** | Hoarseness of voice and V. cord paralysis<br>Extra pyramidal signs with severe autonomic features. | |
| **Sprengel's Syndrome** | Skeletal deformities<br>Scapula lies at an abnormally high level and is distorted and hypoplastic in shape<br>Cervical rib, Absence or malformation of ribs, Spina bifida, Hemivertebrae, Shortened humerus or clavicle and defect in regional muscle (Trapezius). | |

(Contd.......)

## NAMED SYNDROMES (Contd....)

| *Name* | *Symptoms & Signs* | *Treatment* |
|---|---|---|
| **Stevens-Johnson Syndrome** | Pain during swallowing and Fever<br>Severe stomatitis-ulcerative lesions<br>Purulent conjunctivitis<br>Acute febrile reaction. | |
| **Sturge-Weber Syndrome** | Vascular naevi (haemangiomas) along the course of superior and middle branches of trigeminal nerve<br>Glaucoma on same side<br>Haemangiomas of Pia mater. | |
| **Subclavian Steal Syndrome** | Vertigo which is more aggravated by neck twisting. | |
| **Tapia's Syndrome** | Hoarseness of voice and difficulty in speaking.<br>Paralysis of larynx and tongue. | Treat the cause |
| **Taysach's Syndrome** | Ear discharge, Visual disturbances and Jews are usually affected.<br>Amourotic idiocy, Cherry red macula., Otorrhoea, Progressive mental impairment ending in absolute idiocy, Progressive paralysis of wholebody, Progressive dimunition in vision ending in absolute blindness, Optic atrophy, Cherry red spots near macula, Nystagmus and Hyperacusis. | No certain treatment, some patients temporarily respond to corticosteroids. |

(Contd.......)

## NAMED SYNDROMES (Contd....)

| *Name* | *Symptoms & Signs* | *Treatment* |
|---|---|---|
| **Treacher-Collins Syndrome or (Franceschetti Zwahlen Syndrome)** | Aural abnormalities in the form of anotia or micro-otia and Deafness.<br>Underdeveloped lower half of face, especially manidble and maxilla,<br>Notched lower eye lid, called Coloboma<br>Poorly developed eye lashes (No eye lashes in medial 2/3rd of lower eyelid).<br>Microtia or anotia<br>Especially the maxilla and mandible<br>External auditory canal atresia and middle ear abnormalities<br>Abnormal prolongation of hair line on the cheeck<br>Antimongoloid eyes. | Plastic surgery of ears and mandible |
| **Trotter's Syndrome** | Deafness, Nasal twang of voice and Facial pain.<br>Soft palate paralysis on ipsilateral side, with curtain movement of palate.<br>Conductive deafness due to eustachian tube obstruction.<br>Facial neuralgia due to involvement of maxillary division of trigeminal nerve. | Radiotherapy. |
| **Turner's Syndrome** | Short neck and Absence of secondary sexual characters.<br>Sexual infantalism, Cubitus vulgus and Short webbed neck. | |

(Contd.......)

## NAMED SYNDROMES (Contd....)

| *Name* | *Symptoms & Signs* | *Treatment* |
|---|---|---|
| **Usher's Syndrome** | Deafness, Visual disturbances in the form of night blindness.<br>Perceptive deafness and Retinitis pigmentosa. | Hearing aids. |
| **Vander Hoeve-de Kleyn Syndrome** | Deafness, Osteogenesis imperfecta, Blue sclerotics<br>Otosclerotic deafness and repeated fractures of bones.<br>Otosclerotic deafness, Brittle bones. | Stapedectomy and Hearing aids. |
| **Vernet's Syndrome** | Signs and symptoms same as Schmidt's syndrome associated with diminution of taste over posterior third of tongue and loss of pharyngeal sensation.<br>Hoarseness of voice<br>Nasal twang with regurgitation<br>Diminution of taste over posterior 2/3rd of tongue. | Treat the cause<br>Radiotherapy in neoplastic lesions and surgical intervention in inflammatory lesions. |
| **Villaret's Syndrome** | It is same as Vernet's syndrome but is also associate with Horner's syndrome and hence its features are 9, 10, 11th & 12th nerve paralysis (spinal part). | Excision with radiotherapy. |
| **Vogt-Koyanagi-Harada Syndrome** | Deafness, Pain along the distribution of nerve<br>Patchy loss of hair and white patches on skins.<br>Perceptive deafness, neuralgia, Alopecia areata, Vitiligo and whitening of eye lashes. | Carbamazapine for neuralgic pain and hearing aids for deafness. |
| **von Willebrand's Syndrome** | Epistaxis and prolonged bleeding from minor injuries.<br>Purpuric spots and prolonged bleeding time. | Replacement of blood with fresh blood or with purified factor VIII.<br>Aminocaproic acid may also be helpful. |

(Contd.......)

## NAMED SYNDROMES (Contd....)

| *Name* | *Symptoms & Signs* | *Treatment* |
|---|---|---|
| **Waarden Burg's Syndrome (1851)** | Deafness<br>Hypertelorism (Broad nasal root)<br>Congenital perceptive deafness<br>Heterochromia iridis<br>Frontal bosses<br>White fore lock<br>Hypertrichosis of medial portion of eyebrows. | |
| **Wallenbarg's Syndrome (Autosomal dominant)** | Dysphagia, Vertigo, Diplopia, Imbalance, Nystagmus and Muscular paralysis. | Treat the cause. |
| **Wallenburg's Syndrome (Lateral medullary syndrome)** | Severe paroxysm of vertigo with vomiting. Deafness and Neurological signs due to medullary infarction. | Anticoagulants |
| **Wernick's Syndrome** | Vertigo and Pain on moving the eyeball. Nystagmus, Ophthalmoplegia and Ataxia. | Thiamine in large doses. |
| **Whistling face Syndrome** | Microstorne, flattended mid face as in whistling, deep seated eyes, coloboma, alterations of nasal wings, kyphocoliosis, talipes equinovarus, ulnar deviation of fingers. | |
| **Wildervanck's Syndrome** | Short neck and Diplopia.<br>Cervical dysostosis of Klippel-syndrome<br>Retraction of eye and Sixth nerve palsy. | |

# MISCELLANEOUS

## NECK MASS

A. ***Congenital cystic mass of the neck :*** Are usually painless insensitive and slow growing. Some may be present at birth, others appear at a later stage.

1. *Thyro-glossal cyst :* Commonest midline mass, located in the front of the neck close to the hyoid bone. It results from the anomalous presence of median thyroid diverticulum.

   *Treatment :*Complete excision of the duct upto foramen caecum including the body of the hyoid bone.

2. *Branchial cleft cyst :* Commonest cystic lateral neck mass along the anterior border of sternomastoid muscle. It represents the cervical sinus of His and adjacent 2nd or 3rd branchial cleft and pouches. It is a painless, smooth, cystic mass appearing in 2nd or 3rd decade. Sometimes present as a sinus tract along the anterior border of sternomastoid muscle.

   *Treatment :*—Complete excision of the tract upto the pharynx.

3. *Cystic Hygroma :* Is rare and occurs usually in infancy in the posterior triangle. It is lymphangioma of vestigial lymph channel—unilocular or multilocular.

4. *Laryngocele*

5. *Dermoids :* Can occur anywhere along the line of fusion. Treatment is excision.

B. ***Skin and associated subcutaneous mass :***

Sebaceous cyst is the commonest. Neurofibroma, lipoma, melanoma etc. are some other lesions that can occur anywhere in the neck.

C. ***Salivary gland mass***

D. ***Thyroid mass :*** Commonest presentation is simple goitre. Other include thyroiditis, thyroid nodule, toxic goitre, malignant tumour etc. Malignant tumour is often diagnosed by rapid growth, involvement of recurrent laryngeal nerve, dysphagia and respiratory distress.

Student should be able to diagnose thyroid mass (by upward and downward movement with deglutition).

E. ***Primary tumours of neck structure :***

1. Arises from chemoreceptor tissues around carotid bulb and present the histological picture of nonchromaffin paraganglioma. It is benign, pulsatile, firm, slow growing tumour in the carotid triangle.

   *Treatment :* Surgical excision, though often difficult.

2. *Neurogenic tumours :* Neuro-fibroma, Schwannoma, vagal body tumour, etc.

   *Treatment :* Complcte excision.

3. *Branchogenic carcinoma :* Rare, arises from branchial sinus remnant.

F. ***Lymph node mass :***

1. *Infected (Septic) adenitis :* Enlarged jugulo-digastric node (tonsillar) is due to tonsillitis. Other pharyngeal lymphoid tissue inflammation can produce cervical adenitis in upper deep cervical chain and also posterior triangle. Infected lesion of facio-maxillary region and head and neck can produce secondary enlarged tender node in the draining cervical area.

   *Treatment* is of the primary lesion.

2. *Tubercular adenitis :* is very common involving upper deep cervical chain and posterior triangle. They are usually primary—caused by bovine type of the tuberculosis through pharyngeal lymphoid tissue. In supra-clavicular and lower cervical group it may be secondary to pulmonary Koch's periadenitis is characteristic. Sinus formation is uncommon with advancement of drugs and early treatment.

*Diagnosis* is confirmed by gland biopsy and histopathological examination.

*Treatment :* Appropriate antitubercular therapy. In localised lesion, subsequent excision may be necessary.

3. *Syphilitic lymphadenitis :* Rare now-a-days.
4. *Lymphomas :* May be part of systemic disease. They involve neck lymph nodes as well as tonsils, nasopharynx and salivary glands. They are firm, rubbery in consistency—either Hodgkin or Non-Hodgkin's variety (Follicular lymphoma, histiocytic lymphoma etc.).

   *Treatment :* is irradiation combined with chemotherapy.
5. *Metastatic nodes :* From primary head and neck malignant tumours — commonly pharyngeal and laryngeal lesions. Sometimes the primary site of malignancy may be silent or unknown, e.g. (i) Nasopharynx; (ii) Vallecula ; (iii) Pyriform sinus; (iv) Epiglottis—near laryngeal tubercle; (v) Bronchogenic; (vi) Upper oesophagus (vii) Stomach (Virchow's); (viii) Breast ; (ix) Testis, etc.

   *Treatment :* A thorough effort is made to detect the primary. Treatment depends on site—varying from radiotherapy, radical surgery and chemotherapy in some cases.

## TRACHEA

* Trachea is membrao-cartilaginous tube—10-11.5 cm in length in adult.
* Extends from 6th cervical vertebra to 5th thoracic vertebra.
* Trachea comprises 16 to 20 incomplete rings of cartilage and upper 6 or 7 being in the neck.
* Tracheal mucosa is lined by ciliated columnar epithelium.

## TRACHEOBRONCHIAL TREE

*Endoscopic Anatomy :*

* Bifurcation of tracheal is 25 cm from incisor teeth & at the level of upper border of 5th thoracic vertebra.

* Right main bronchus has large diameter, shorter & more vertical than left (foreign bodies have tendency to enter into right main bronchus).
* Left main bronchus is narrower, larger & more horizontal than right.

## OESOPHAGUS

* Oesophagus developed from primitive foregut.
* 25 cm long muscular oesophagus extends from lower border of cricoid cartilage above at the level of 6th cervical vertebra to cardiac orifice of stomach below at the level of 11th thoracic vertebra.
* Oesophageal constrictions are at 15 cm to 25 cm from incisor teeth.
  * At 25 cm—oesophagus is crossed by aortic arch & left main bronchus
  * At 40 cm — oesophagus pierces diaphragm (at 10th thoracic vertebra level).
* Oesophagus is lined by stratified squamous epithelium
* *Arterial supply*
  * Inferior thyroid artery (cervical part).
  * Descending thoracic aorta (cervical part)
  * Left gastric artery (abdominal part)
* *Venous drainage :*
  * Inferior thyroid vein (cervical part).
  * Azygous vein (thoracic part)
  * Left gastric vein (abdominal part).
* *Nerve supply*—Parasympathetic (vagi) & sympathetic trunk.
* *Lymphatic drainage*—Posterior mediastinal lymph nodes.

***Constrictions of the oesophagus :*** There are four constrictions :

1. At the pharyngo-oesophageal junction formed by cricopharyngeal sphincter (part of inferior constrictor muscle) at the level of sixth cervical vertebra (15 cm from upper incisor).
2. At the level of arch of the aorta—4th dorsal vertebra (25 cm from upper incisor).
3. At the crossing of the left bronchus—5th dorsal vertebral (27 cm from upper incisor).
4. As it passes through diaphragm (10th dorsal vertebra).

# INDICATIONS OF TRACHEOSTOMY

A. ***To relieve respiratory obstruction :*** Which is evident by supra-clavicular, supra-sternal and intercostal retraction; inspiratory stridor; restlessness; apprehension; pallor and cyanosis (late) & exhaustion.

I. *Intrinsic causes :*

a) Congenital : Laryngeal web, laryngeal stenosis, tracheo-oesophageal fistula etc.

1. *Traumatic :*
   a) Inhalation of fumes.
   b) Swallowing corrosives
   c) Instrumentation, particularly in children.
2. *Foreign body :* impacted in the larynx
3. *Infective :*
   a) Acute laryngo-tracheo-bronchitis.
   b) Diphtheretic laryngitis
   c) Oedema larynx
   d) Acute epiglottitis.
4. *Paralytic :*
   a) Bilateral recurrent laryngeal nerve paralysis.
   b) Fixation of the arytenoids in rheumatoid arthritis.
5. *Allergic :* Angio-neurotic oedema.
6. *Neoplastic :*
   a) *Benign :* Multiple papillomatosis of the larynx.
   b) *Malignant :* Carcinoma of the larynx and pharynx causing dyspnoea.

II. *Extrinsic causes :*

1. Traumatic : External injury to the larynx, cut-throat wound etc.
2. Pressure from outside : Malignant thyroid, or any other tumour in the neck causing pressure to the larynx and trachea.
3. Paralytic :
   a) Post-thyroidectomy : Injury to both recurrent laryngeal nerves.
   b) Cancer oesophagus : Involving recurrent laryngeal nerve.
4. Infective : Ludwig's angina.

B. ***For assisted respiration and protection to the tracheobronchial tree:***

1. *Lesions of higher centre, unconscious patients or comatose patients :* Head injury, cerebro-vascular accidents, encephalitis and other causes of coma of central origin.
2. *Lesions causing depression of respiratory centre :* Bulbar paralysis, barbiturate poisoning and other drug intoxications.
3. *Lesions of anterior horn cells and nerves cotrolling the muscles of respiration :* Poliomyelitis, polyneuritis, cervical spinal injury, myasthenia gravis etc.
4. *Lesions affecting myo-neural junction :* Tetanus
5. *Lesions of the chest wall :* Multiple fracture of ribs, stove-in-chest, flail chest etc.
6. *Lesions of the lungs :* Collapse, fibrosis, emphysema and other chronic obstructive lesion of lungs leading to alveolar hypo-ventilation.
7. Burns of face, neck and chest.

C. ***Planned tracheostomy : To avoid post-operative respiratory complications by aspiration.***

1. In radical operations of the jaw, tongue, pharynx, etc.
2. Operation on the larynx itself such as laryngo-fissure.
3. Facio-maxillary injury and surgery.

D. ***Tracheo-bronchial toilet :*** Emphysema, status asthmaticus, bronchiectasis, etc. with respiratory insufficiency.

***Complications of tracheostomy :***

1. *Immediate :* During the operation or immediately after the operation.
2. *Delayed :* In the post-operative period.
3. *Late :* After few weeks.

1. ***Immediate complications :***

a) *Haemorrhage :* During operation, this primary haemorrhage is due to damage to engorged vessels.

b) *Injury to great vessels :* Carotid artery or jugular vein may be damaged, if one goes on dissecting too laterally instead of keeping in midline.

c) *Injury to nerves* : Recurrent laryngeal nerve may be damaged.

d) *Damage to the apical pleura* : Particularly in children. This will lead to pneumothorax or haemo-pneumothorax causing respiratory distress.

e) *Damage to the cricoid cartilage* : Leads to stenosis later on.

f) *Apnoea* : Sudden apnoea may occur as soon as the trachea is opened due to (i) release of carbon-dioxide which is respiratory stimulant; (ii) carbon-dioxide intoxication of respiratory centre and (iii) relief of hypoxia.

g) *Tracheo-oesophageal fistula* : If the posterior wall is damaged or perforated while incising the tracheal wall, then tracheo-oesophageal fistula may occur endangering the life of the patient.

h) *Aspiration and collapse of the lung.*

i) *Aerophagia in infants.*

2. ***Delayed complications :***

   1. *Surgical emphysema* : Due to light suturing of wound.
   2. *Respiratory tract infection* : Tracheitis, tracheo-bronchitis, pneumonia, atelectasis, lung abscess etc.
   3. *Dysphagia* : Due to lack of positive subglottic pressure in tracheostomy and often due to cuffed tube.
   4. *Reactionary or secondary haemorrhage.*
   5. *Pyo-pneumothorax* : From infection of haemo-pneumothorax.
   6. *Mediastinitis.*
   7. *Pre-tracheal displacement* : The tube may be displaced in the pretracheal space, particularly during changing of the tube.
   8. *Crusting* in trachea.

3. ***Late complications :***

   1. *Laryngeal stenosis* : If cricoid is damaged, then subglottic stenosis occurs.
   2. *Tracheal stenosis* : At the site and distal to tracheostomy.
   3. *Decannulation problem* : Particularly in children.
   4. *Tracheo-cutaneous fistula.*
   5. *Tracheomalacia.*
   6. *Depressed scar.*

***Tracheostomy in infants and children :*** Should be avoided whenever possible :

Special precautions are to be taken to avoid complications :

a) Should be performed after endotracheal intubation or passing a bronchoscope.

b) Low tracheostomy is to be avoided to prevent damage to apical pleura.

c) Incise trachea not too deeply.

d) Minimum excision of cartilage to avoid stenosis and tracheomalacia.

e) Avoid post-operative aerophagia by naso-gastric feeding.

f) Prevent lower respiratory tract infection by aseptic care and antibiotic.

g) Should be prepared for decannulation problem.

---

## ANATOMY OF THE LARYNX

---

***Embryology of Larynx :***

* Hypobranchial eminence or copula is formed on the floor of the primitive pharynx.
* Thyroid cartilage—developes from ventral ends of 4th visceral arch.
* Cricoid cartilage—from 6th arch.
* Arytenoid cartilage—from 6th arch.
* Epiglottis—from 4th arch
* Sphincter & dilator muscles of larynx develops from mesoderm of 6th arch (inner constrictor layer of primitive pharynx) & Tensor muscles develops from outer ring musculature of primitive pharynx.
* Larynx lies infront of laryngopharynx from 3rd to 6th cervical vertebrae.

---

*Regions of Larynx :*

*Supraglottis :*

* *Epilarynx (including marginal zone)*
  * Posterior surface of the suprahyoid epiglottis including the tip
  * Aryepiglottic folds
  * Arytenoids
* *Supraglottis (excluding epilarynx)*
  * Infrahyoid epiglottis
  * Ventricular bands
  * Ventricular cavities

*Glottis :*

* Vocal cords
* Anterior commissure
* Posterior commissure

*Subglottis :*

* Walls of the subglottis.

***Cartilages of the larynx***

It consists of :

1. Unpaired—

   a) Thyroid b) Cricoid c) Epiglottis.

2. Paired :

   a) Arytenoids b) Corniculates c) Cuneiforms.

***Muscles of the larynx :***

1. *Extrinsic :*

   (i) Sterno-thyroid (ii) Thyro-hyoid
   (iii) Stylo-pharyngeus (iv) Palato-pharyngeus and
   (v) Inferior constrictor of the pharynnx.

2. *Intrinsic :* Only inter-arytenoid is single and others are paired.

   (i) Abductor of the vocal cords : Crico-arytenoid posterior. This is also called "*Safety muscle* of the larynx". This comes into action during respiration.

(ii) Adductors : Crico-arytenoid lateralis; Inter-arytenoid; thyro-arytenoid; and crico-thyroid (partly). Adductors come into action during phonation.

(iii) Tensors and adductors : Crico-thyroid, vocalis and thyro-arytenoid.

***Interior of the larynx :***

Extends from the inlet of the larynx to the lower border of the cricoid cartilage. This is divided into 3 parts by two folds : false vocal cords (ventricular band) and true vocal cords.

1. *Vestibule* is the space between the inlet of the larynx above and the false vocal cords below.
2. *Ventricle of the larynx b* is the recess between the false and true vocal cords. The saccule is a conical pouch which ascends from ant. part of the vestibule.

   ***The glottis*** (Rima glottidis) is the interval between the true vocal cords in the anterior 2/3rd and vocal process in the posterior 1/3rd. Average length in adult is 2.5 cm.
3. *Subglottic space* lies below the true vocal cords and upto the lower border of the cricoid cartilage

***Mucous membrane of the larynx :***

Upper part of epiglottis. A.E. folds and vocal cords are lined by stratified squamous epithelium. Remaining part is lined by respiratory epithelium.

***Nerve supply of the larynx :***

1. *Superior laryngeal nerve :* Supplies sensory fibres to the inner surface above true vocal cords. Its external branch supplies the crico-thyroid muscle.
2. *Recurrent laryngeal nerve :* Supplies all the intrinsic muscles of the larynx except the crico-thyroid and sensory fibres to the larynx below the vocal cords.

***Lymphatic drainage :***

The true vocal cords are devoid of lymphatic vessels

1. *Supraglottic space :* Drains into upper deep cervical nodes which lie on the internal jugular vein, and pre-epiglottic nodes.
2. *Subglottic space :* Drains into pretracheal, prelaryngeal and lower deep cervical nodes.

## SYMPTOMS & SIGNS

* *Voice strain*—Larynx shows—glottis open
* Appearance of bowing of vocal cords is due to thyro-arytenoid muscle weakness.
* *Triangular gap posteriorly*—is due to interarytenoid muscle weakness.
* *Key hole apearance*—if both thyroarytenoid & interarytenoid muscles weakness.
* Acid laryngitis—Hypertrophy of interarytenoid area (pachydermia) presents as hoarseness of voice & shows 'contact ulcers'.
* *Vocal nodules or Singer's nodes or Screamer's nodes*—Hoarse voice & vocal cords shows bilateral, small & greyish—white nodules & are located at the junction of anterior third & posterior two-thirds of glottis.
* Dysphonia plicae ventricularis—Phonation with false vocal cords instead of true cords, patient produces 'duct' like sound.
* Laryngomalacia—(Congenital laryngeal stridor)—Stridor soon after birth (croaking & in inspiratory phase) inspiratory stridor without horasenes.
* Laryngeal web—Hoarseness, insipiratory stridor, dyspnoea on exertion.
* Singer's nodes—Hoarseness, vocal fatigue, bilateral symmetrical nodules on cords.
* contact 'ulcer of vocal cords—Throat discomfort, huskiness, vocal fatigue, referred otalgia & 'kiss ulcer'.
* Acute epiglottitis —Dyspnoea & pain on swallowing.
* Acute laryngo-tracheobronchitis—Hard, dry, croupy cough & hoarseness, pyrexia, dyspnoea & cyanosis, tenacious exudation & crusting, oedema of larynx and atelectasis.
* **Vocal cord position, opening**

  **Position vocal cord opening**

  Median—Both cords in midline

  Paramedian—3.5 mm

  Intermediate—7 mm

  Slight abduction—14 mm

  Full abduction—18-19 mm

## COMMONEST SITE OF LESION

| *Laryngeal lesion* | *Commonest site* |
|---|---|
| Laryngeal atresia | Subglottis |
| Congenital laryngeal web | Between vocal cords (always in anterior part) |
| Congenital syphilis & chronic hypetrophic laryngitis | Supraglottis & Glottis |
| Tuberculosis | Posterior part of glottis |
| Primary & secondary syphilis | Anterior half of glottis |
| Gumma | Anywhere |
| Lupus vulgaris | Epiglottis |
| Leprosy | Epiglottis & Aryepiglottic folds |
| Scleroma | Subglottis |
| Laryngeal cleft | Posterior part |
| Congenital true retention cyst | Supraglottis |
| Haemangioma & retention cyst | Supraglottis |
| Haemangioma & Lymphangioma | Subglottis & vocal cord |
| Chondroma | Cricoid cartilage |
| Fibroma | Over dorsum of vocal cord |
| Papilloma | Free edge of vocal cord |

## VOCAL CORDS PARALYSIS

A. ***Unilateral***

1. **Left recurrent laryngeal nerve paralysis**—more common.

   I. **Causes in the chest** :

      a) Carcinoma bronchus
      b) Mediastinal growth or metastatic nodes.
      c) Carcinoma oesophagus.
      d) Enlarged heart (mitral stenosis).
      e) Aortic aneurysm.
      f) Following "Patent ductus arteriosus" operation
      g) Pulmonary tuberculosis and fibrosis.

II. Causes in the neck :

a) Carcinoma thyroid

b) Following thyroid surgery

c) Penetrating wound

d) Malignant metastasis

e) Cancer oesophagus

III. Idiopathic

2. Right recurrent laryngeal nerve paralysis : Causes are mainly in the neck as its course is in the neck only :

a) Causes in the neck are same as on the left side. Right nerve is more commonly involved in thyroid surgery.

b) Apical tuberculosis

c) Pancoast tumour

B. ***Bilateral Paralysis***

1. Abductor :

a) Idiopathic

b) Malignant disease of the thyroid

c) Thyroid surgery

d) Carcinoma of the oesophagus

e) Cut-throat injury

f) Peripheral neuritis

2. Adductor paralysis is mainly functional or hysterical. This is commonly seen in young girls or women with psychological background.

3. Total paralysis is seen in viral neuritis, peripheral neuritis etc. Here superior laryngeal nerve is also involved.

# HOARSENESS OF VOICE AND DIAGNOSIS

***Aetiology :***

1. *Laryngeal causes :*

   a) Congenital

   b) Traumatic

      1. External : strangulation, injury neck, etc.

      2. Internal : instrumentation, fumes, operative, etc.

   c) Inflammatory :

      1. Acute : acute laryngitis, oedema larynx etc.

      2. Chronic : chronic laryngitis, singer's node, etc.

      3. Specific : T.B. syphilis, etc.

   d) Neoplastic :

      (i) Benign : papilloma, vocal nodule, fibroma, angioma etc.

      (ii) Malignant : carcinoma commonly

   e) Paralytic : motor paralysis

   f) Allergic : angio-neurotic oedema

   g) Functional or hysterical

   h) Miscellaneous : dysphonia plica ventricularis

2. ***Pharyngeal & Oesophageal causes :***

   a) Hypopharyngeal carcinoma involving larynx.

   b) Pharyngeal pouch

   c) Carcinoma oesophagus

3. ***General causes :*** Myxoedema, renal or cardiac oedema, other causes of anasarca, etc.

4. ***Neck (including thyroid disease) and mediastinal causes :*** Leading to laryngeal nerve paralysis.

* **Abnormalities of tongue size**

**Large tongue**

Hypothyroidism
Trisomy-21
Beckwith-Wiedemann syndrome
Tumor
Cyst

**Small tongue**

Aglossia
Hypoglossia

* **Epiglottic and Aryepiglottic fold enlargement**

Epiglottitis
Angioneurotic edema
Corrosive burns
Face and neck edema
Tumor
Aryepiglottic fold cyst
Sarcoidosis
Haemarrhage (hemophilia)
Radiation

* **Vocal Cord Abnormalities**

**Indistinct, fuzzy on lateral view**

Croup
Paralysis
Trauma
Storage diseases
Lipoid proteinosis

**Bilateral cord thickening and/or fixation**

Croup
Trauma (latrogenic)
Paralysis
Epiglottitis

Trauma (non-iatrogenic)

Laryngeal web

Storage diseases

Lipoid proteinosis

**Unilateral thickening and/or fixation**

Paralysis

Iatrogenic trauma

Subglottic hemangioma

Laryngeal web (unilateral)

**Nodules**

Papillomatosis

Postintubation granuloma

Benign and malignant tumors

* **Subglottic tracheal narrowing circumferential**

Croup

Subglottic stenosis

Paradoxic collapse with other glottic obstruction

**Eccenteric**

Subglottic hemangioma

Post-tracheostomy fibrosis

Intratracheal thyroid

Subglottic mucocele

Histiocytoma

Papilloma

Intratracheal thymus

# AIRWAY OBSTRUCTION IN CHILDREN

| *Site* | *Voice* | *Stridor* | *Retractions* | *Mouth* | *Feeding* | *Cough* |
|---|---|---|---|---|---|---|
| Nasal nasopharynx | Hyponasal | Sonorous inspiratory | Entire chest esp. when asleep | Open | Poor choking and aspiration | Normal |
| Oropharynx | Muffled | Inspiratory coarse, snore | Entire chest | Open | Difficult saliva pooling | Normal |
| Supraglottis | Muffled | Inspiratory sonorous | None until late | Open, tripod | impossible | Wet |
| Subglottis | Hoarse | Inspirations early, expirations late | Early xiphoid and intercostal late whole | Closed alar flaring | Normal or dysphagia | Barking |
| Tracheo-bronchial | Normal | Expiratory wheezing to and fro | Xiphoid and sternal prolonged, exp hyperinflation | Closed, alar flaring | Normal | Brassy |

# TREATMENT OF CHOICE

**Voice problems**

* Voice strain—Total voice rest for 1-2 weeks.
* Acid laryngitis—Histamine ($H_2$) antagonists & antacids at night.
* Very small vocal nodules—Speech therapy.
* Vocal nodules with hoarse voice—Removal of vocal nodules by direct laryngoscopy (using microsurgical techniques) + Followed by speech therapy.
* Dysphonia plicae ventricularis—Speech therapy.

**Subglottic stenosis**

* Congenital subglottic stenosis in children—Conservation treatment (SOS—airway threatening—tracheostomy).
* Children with significant subglottic stenosi—Tracheostomy (between 5th & 6th tracheal rings).

**Laryngeal stridor**

* Laryngeal Atresia recognised at birth—Tracheostomy.
* Congenital medium sized webs—Removal by microlaryngoscopy + injection of steroids at anterior end of vocal cords (to prevent adhesions).
* Laryngomalacia (congenital laryngeal stridor)—Symptomatic with ressurance to the parents + Early antibiotic therapy (for upper respiratory tract infections).
* Foreign bodies in the larynx —(Removal through laryngoscope under careful general anaesthesia).
* Acute epiglottitis—Most oxygen + Sedation + Chloramphenicol (antibiotic of choice) & SOS—Suction & Special nursing of the child.

**Laryngeal infections**

* Acute laryngitis—Bed rest + Voice rest + steam inhalation with menthol or tincture of benzoin (SOS—if pain—salicylic acid analgesics & if secondary infection—Amoxycillin (drug of choice).
* Chronic laryngitis—Voice rest + Speech therapy + Avoidance of pollutants + Local application of glucose in glycerin or oil of pine.

* Chronic laryngitis with oedema & hypertrophic laryngitis—Vocal cord stripping through endoscopy.
* Perichondritis of larynx —Ampicillin + Diuretics.
* Perichondritis of larynx with oedema & useless 6 months after radiation therapy—total laryngectomy (even if biopsy is -ve for residual cancer).
* Candidiasis of the larynx—Resolves with cessation of steroid inhaler.
* *Arthritis of the cricoarytenoid joint—*
    * Acute phase—Symptomatic treatment (analgesics) & SOS—steroids.
    * Chronic phase with joint fixed in adduction position with good voice—No treatment (SOS—chronic phase—Cordopexy or arytenoid operation).

**Rare laryngeal tumours**

* Laryngocele—Removal of laryngocele sac.
* Laryngeal cyst (Supraglottic cysts)—Uncap cyst through direct laryngoscopy (permanent marsupilisation).
* Vocal cord polyp—Removal by microlaryngoscopy.
* Prolapse of the ventricle of the larynx—Endoscopic removal of the medial portion of projection (Diathermy puncture results in fibrosis & prevents recurrence).
* Intubation granuloma of the larynx—Removal locally along with infected cartilage (to prevent recurrence).

**Cancer of the larynx**

* Carcinoma-in-situ of the vocal cord—Repeated vocal cord stripping.
* Carcinoma-in-situ with areas of invasion cancer of larynx—Radiotherapy.

*Supraglottic cancer :*

* Patients with metastatic nodes—Surgery.
* T1 NO & T2 NO Supraglottic tumours—radiotherapy
* T3 NO & T4 No Supraglottic tumours—Surgery.
* T1N1 or T2N1 supraglottic tumours—Supraglottic laryngectomy.

*Glottic Cancer :*

* T1 Glottic cancer—Radiotherapy
* T1 Glottic cancer with recurrence—surgery (either Haemilaryngectomy or total laryngectomy).

*Transglottic cancer :*

* Transglottic tumour with palpable cervical nodes—total laryngectomy with radical neck dissection.
* Transglottic tumours with no nodes palpable—Radiotherapy (primary treatment).
* Recurrence after primary radiotherapy with swollen larynx—total laryngectomy.

*Subglottic cancer :*

* Primary treatment of subglottic cancer—Primary radiotherapy
* Recurrence of subglottic cancer—total laryngectomy + Removal of paratracheal nodes.
* Large subglottic tumour presenting with respiratory obstruction—Emergency laryngectomy.

**Vocal cord paralysis :**

I. *Unilateral adductor paralysis :*

* Unilateral adductor paralysis with a large shift requirement—Implant procedure (Ishiki laryngoplasty).
* Bilateral adductor paralysis with oedematous & infected larynx & upper trachea (severe situation—total laryngectomy).

II. *Bilateral adductor paralysis with oedema*—Total laryngectomy.

III. *Unilateral abductor paralysis*—No treatment.

IV. *Bilateral abductor paralysis* (functional aphonia)—Reassurance, psychotherapy.

***Indications for Laryngofissure :***

* Removal of small intralaryngeal tumours.
* Excision of webs or strictures.
* Submucous excision of one vocal cord.
* Removal of impacted foreign body.

***Indications for Partial Laryngectomy :***

* Lateral partial laryngectomy—for limited cordal tumours.
* Frontolateral partial laryngectomy—for glottic tumours (which cross the anterior commissure).
* Supraglottic partial laryngectomy—for lesions of the infrahyoid epiglottis & adnexae (to spare vocal cords).

***Indication for total laryngectomy :***

* Advanced carcinomas of larynx.

***Laryngectomy***

*Indications :*

1. Carcinoma of one vocal cord which has spread round the anterior commissure and involved the anterior third of other cord.
2. Carcinoma of ventricular band.
3. Subglottic carcinoma
4. Failed irradiation
5. Radio-resistant tumour.

*Types : Total and partial*

A. *Total* is often associated with block dissection of neck. Whole of Larynx with hyoid bone is mobilised and excised along with few rings of trachea. Thyroid lobe is often excised on th side of lesion. Permanent tracheostomy is performed. Pharynx and oesophagus are repaired carefully.

B. *Partial Laryngectomy :* This is conservative form of surgery where the growth is localised, with a view to preserve the functional element of voice box i.e. voice and protective functions.

*Different types :*

1. Laryngo-fissure (Lateral partial laryngectomy) : Whole of affected vocal cord, vocal process of arytenoid, deep tissue and overlying thyroid cartilage with internal perichondrium are removed by splitting thyroid cartilage.
2. Supraglottic partial laryngectomy : Supraglottic part of larynx is removed and lower half of larynx is anastomosed with pharynx.

   Associated block dissection is often performed.

3. Hemilaryngectomy (vertical partial laryngectomy) : One half of larynx is removed and the resultant gap is closed by strap muscles fashioned to form a false vocal cord.

## INDICATIONS FOR TONSILLECTOMY

* Recurrent episodes of acute tonsillitis (5/year/fo at least one year)
* One episode of peritonsillar abscess (Quinsy).
* Febrile convulsions.
* Carrier states (e.g diphtheria or β hemolytic streptococci).
* Suspected malignancy (eg lymphoma).
* Chronic tonsillitis.
* As part of another surgical procedure (e.g. UVPP or transirak resection of the styloid process).
* Gross obstruction (e.g. obstructive sleep apnoea syndrome).

## INDICATIONS FOR ADENOIDECTOMY

* Nasal obstruction
* Chronic infective rhino-sinusitis
* Recurrent acute otitis media
* Recurrent middle ear effusion (OME)
* Obstructive sleep apnoea

## CONTRAINDICATIONS TO TONSILLECTOMY AND ADENOIDECTOMY

* Recurrent upper resp. tract infection
* Bleeding disorders
* Oral contraceptive pill
* Cleft palate and submucous cleft
* Epidemics (Polio meningitis)

# IMPORTANT SIGNS AND SYMPTOMS

## MOUTH

* ***Oral Pigmentation***

  *White*

  Moniliasis, pearly white

  Lichen planus; pearly white

  Red

  pernicious anaemia tongue; red and smooth

  vitamin B deficiency : magenta tongue

  polycythaemia: blue-red

  *Yellow*

  herpangina : yellow grey

  syphilitic rhagades: golden

  cadmium poisoning : golden gingivitis

  *Black*

  Addison's disease: black patches

  Peutz-Jegher's syndrome : black

  bismuth }
  mercury } poisoning blue-black gums
  lead }

* **Helitosis**

  Diet

  Smoker's breath

  Faulty oral hygiene

  Continued mouth breathing

  Acute ulcerative gingivitis

  Chronic periodonititis

  Infected tooth socket

  Pericoronitis

  Descending pharyngeal exudate from infected sinus

  Tonsillitis

Bronchiectasis

Lung abscess

Rare

pharyngeal pouch

oesophageal diverticula

* ***Gum hyperplasia***

Physiological

In mouth breathers during childhood pregnancy

Pathological

Long-term therapy with phenytoin (anticonvulsant)

Chronic infection of gums ill-fitting dentures vitamin C deficiency acute myeloblastic leukaemia.

* ***Bleeding Gums***

Bleeding gums in systemic disease scurvy

associated with purpura

any thrombocytopenia

Platelet dysfunction including acute leukaemia

bleeding diathesis associated with plasma coagulation factor deficiencies.

* ***Bilateral parotid gland enlargement***

Mumps

Infectious mononucleosis

Mickulicz's disease

Sarcoidosis

Sjogren's syndrome

Chronic pancreatitis

Cirrhosis

## NOSE

* ***Nasal collapse***

Infection

syphilis

- congenital
- tertiary

yaws

leprosy

cutaneous leishmaniasis

blastomycosis

phycomycosis

Vasculitis (collagen disorders)

- Wegener's granuloma
- lethal midline granuloma } are causes
- polyarteritis nodosa
- systemic lupus erythematosus
- rheumatoid arthritis
- scleroderma
- psoriatic arthritis
- Malignancy : Carcinoma of the nose and nasopharynx

## THROAT

* ***Membranes in throat***

Moniliasis

Infectious mononucleosis

Diphtheria

Vincent's angina

Acute leukaemia

Agranulocytosis

(Haemolytic streptococcal infection : follicular patches)

* ***Necrotizing Infection of the External Auditory Canal***

(Malignant's otitis externa)

Predisposing conditions

- diabetes mellitus
- old age
- pseudomonas pyocyanea infection
- minor trauma to external auditory canal blood dyscrasia

Differential diagnosis

- severe pyogenic infection
- otomycosis
- tuberculosis of the ear
- carcinoma of the ear
- eosinophilic granuloma
- Wegener's granuloma
- tumours of the glomus jugulare

* ***Non-suppurative Otitis Media, 'Glue Ear', Mucinous or Serous Otitis Media***

Due to dysfunction of Eustachian tubes ass. with deficient palatal musculature

in cleft palate<br>
enlarged adenoids<br>
chronic sinusitis<br>
} aggravated by upper respiratory tract infections

allergic rhinitus

* ***Acute sensorineural deafness***

Central

- encephalitis
- meningomyelitis
- pontine glioma
- concussion
- psychogenic of sudden onset

Cochlear

viral

herpes zoster, measles, mumps vascular lesions

suppurative labyrinthitis

leptomeningitis

cochlear otosclerosis

tuberculous meningitis
tumours
syphilitic meningitis
autoimmune disease
arachnoiditis
ototoxic drugs e.g. gentamycin, streptomycin
angle meningioma
tomycin Results of trauma
Meniere's disease
concussion
late syphilis
labyrinthine window rupture
Retrocochlear
stapes fracture
multiple sclerosis
fractured otic capsule
acoustic neuroma
decompression deafness
meningitis